TRIP REPORTS

Rich Haridy is a freelance writer and journalist based in Melbourne, Australia. After spending 15 years playing various roles in the psychedelic underground, he watched this previously taboo field come out of the shadows and into mainstream culture. In 2016, he started following the renaissance of psychedelic science as a journalist. His writing can be found in *Nature, Salon, Cosmos Magazine, New Atlas* and *The Best Australian Science Writing* 2024 and 2025.

'*Trip Reports* is a mind-expanding journey through Australia's unique and little-known history of psychedelic discovery and its current world-leading therapeutic initiatives. Across its deeply informed, lucid and highly readable narrative, Rich Haridy untangles the mysteries and debates that range across the spectrum from plant evolution to pharmacology to mental health. His conclusions challenge the currently hyped model of therapy and point towards radical new horizons.'

Mike Jay, author of *Psychonauts: Drugs and the Making of the Modern Mind*

'An intelligently critical and up-to-date discussion of the psychedelic field. *Trip Reports* is an even-handed and evidence-based exploration of psychedelics and their potential, while avoiding the hype.'

Lynne Malcolm, author of *All in the Mind*

'A cool, exacting look at psychedelics that cuts through the noise to bring clarity and nuance to a rapidly evolving field.'

Alison Pouliot, author of *Underground Lovers: Encounters with fungi and Wild Mushrooming*

'Like the internet revolution, the psychedelic renaissance is just a story: a narrative that is being co-opted by capitalism, individualism and pharmaceutical imperialism. It's not too late to retrieve the humanising potential of these substances, but we must begin by taking account of what's really happening here. Rich Haridy combines the rigour of a true journalist with the epistemic modesty of an intellectual in an engaging and necessary read for anyone who hopes for psychedelics to remain truly transformational.'

Douglas Rushkoff, author of *Team Human*

TRIP REPORTS

STORIES FROM AN AUSTRALIAN PSYCHEDELIC RENAISSANCE

RICH HARIDY

NEWSOUTH

UNSW Press acknowledges the Bidjigal people, the Traditional Owners of the unceded territory on which the Randwick and Kensington campuses of UNSW are situated, and recognises the continuing connection to Country and culture. We pay our respects to Elders past and present.

A NewSouth book

Published by
NewSouth Publishing
University of New South Wales Press Ltd
University of New South Wales
Sydney NSW 2052
AUSTRALIA
https://unsw.press/

Our authorised representative in the EU for product safety is Mare Nostrum Group B.V., Doelen 72, 4831 GR Breda, The Netherlands (gpsr@mare-nostrum.co.uk).

First published 2026

NATIONAL LIBRARY OF AUSTRALIA
A catalogue record for this book is available from the National Library of Australia

ISBN 9781761170454 (paperback)
9781761179488 (ebook)
9781761178818 (ePDF)

Cover design Laura Thomas
Cover image iStock/1909988582
Internal design Josephine Pajor-Markus

UNSW
SYDNEY

CONTENTS

INTRODUCTION

Have you heard the story of Albert Hofmann, the Swiss biochemist who accidentally discovered the psychoactive effects of a drug called LSD? Hofmann was working for a company called Sandoz and, in the early 1940s, decided to re-examine some chemicals previously synthesised from a common fungus.

The oft-told story begins on 16 April 1943, when Hofmann was suddenly overcome by an intoxicating dizziness while working in the lab with a substance known as lysergic acid diethylamide (LSD). Suspecting he had accidentally absorbed some of this experimental compound, Hofmann decided to test a tiny dose on himself a few days later.

On 19 April, Hofmann reportedly consumed a quarter of a milligram of LSD. He estimated this miniscule 250-microgram dose would be small enough to establish whether the drug was psychoactive, but he had profoundly underestimated the potency of LSD. About an hour after consuming the drug, he began to feel unsettled. He asked a colleague to help get him home and the pair set out on a 30-minute bicycle journey that subsequently became an iconic birthing moment for 20th-century psychedelic culture.

In his autobiography 35 years later, Hofmann wrote of seeing kaleidoscopic visions, coloured fountains and enjoyable closed-eye hallucinations. He told of how he woke up the next day with a 'sensation of well-being and renewed life'. His breakfast tasted extraordinary and the world glistened in a new light.

The story became a kind of transcendent 'eureka' fable. In 1985, 19 April was branded 'Bicycle Day' by a psychology professor in the United States. Soon after, psychedelic evangelists began their pilgrimage to Switzerland from all corners of the globe to take LSD and re-enact Hofmann's fateful journey. The moment was likened to the detonation of an atomic bomb, with Hofmann the first human to experience an LSD trip, triggering a revolution in Western medicine, science and culture. But the story of Hofmann's first hallucinatory bike ride is, like many origin stories, a mixture of truth and fiction, and embellished over the years to become a grand folk tale.

Historians such as Alan Piper and Mike Jay have since written longer, more complicated stories of Western experimentation with psychedelics, spanning occult uses of mescaline in 1920s London to compellingly conspiratorial descriptions of possible LSD consumption in the 1930s. Mike Jay excavated Hofmann's original 'trip report': the description of that fateful bicycle journey that Hofmann filed to his Sandoz superiors three days after the event. That report, as described by Jay, is quite different from the version in Hofmann's autobiography *LSD: My Problem Child*. 'There are no fantastic images or coloured fountains,' Jay writes. 'It's a gruelling episode that Hofmann experienced as an acute poisoning, with symptoms that were mostly physical and extremely unpleasant. Rather than a psychedelic, he and the visiting doctor compared them to a massive overdose of amphetamines.'[1]

From all primary source reports, that magical bicycle trip was a rather harrowing and mostly uncomfortable experience. Hofmann spoke of dizziness, panic, anxiety, confusion and periods of paralysis. Even the next-day rejuvenation he wrote about decades later was, at the time, described flatly as waking up 'feeling perfectly healthy again, if somewhat weary'.

Hofmann's infamous bicycle trip may be to some degree apocryphal, but it serves as a succinct example of how the stories we tell often shift and transmogrify over time. They become simplified origin stories, blending piecemeal events into a slicker, more singular narrative. There isn't anything inherently wrong with this process. This is the nature of storytelling, the nature of history-making. We create the narratives that are useful to us.

Over the last decade, one very particular narrative has appeared: 'the psychedelic renaissance'. This story tells of a brave cadre of researchers who risked their professional reputations by investigating the therapeutic potential of psychedelics. From around the early 2010s, a notable shift in the tenor of news reports about psychedelics emerged. For decades these drugs had been regarded in the mainstream as dangerous recreational substances, but now words like 'medicine' and 'therapeutic' were appearing in media reports.[2]

I started working as a science journalist in 2016 and pretty quickly my focus was subsumed by reporting on psychedelics. Having been immersed in psychedelic counterculture throughout my younger years, it felt a little like coming full circle. Discussions I'd had about the weird pharmacology of LSD in 2006 with scientist friends who had only been able to investigate these drugs informally were suddenly at the centre of published articles in serious scientific journals. The psychedelic renaissance had arrived.

I wrote my first big story on the topic in 2017 – a dive into the wave of research turning what had been known as the party drug 'ecstasy' into a legitimate medicine for post-traumatic stress disorder. Over the next few years, I penned dozens more stories on the growth of psychedelic science. Slowly it became apparent to me that the same story was being written by journalists all over the world.

It's a trite saying, but all trite sayings emerge from truth: journalism is the first draft of history. And history requires storytelling. The grand narratives that emerge to dominate the stories we tell solidify through repetition. A very specific story of a psychedelic renaissance had taken shape. And to become a kind of inarguable gospel truth, it needed to be told, and retold, and retold again. So that's what ended up happening. Every media publication on the face of the Earth took their turn doing a psychedelic renaissance story – and they were all similar.

A few years ago I published an article called 'How to Write a Psychedelic Renaissance News Story'.[3] It was a snarky piece of writing, throwing stones at fellow journalists who I'm sure were sincere in trying to do their work and tell the stories they wanted to tell. In hindsight I'm a little embarrassed at how passive aggressive the piece was, but it stemmed from a genuine frustration at finding the same story told over and over and over again.

You see, my problem wasn't that this grand narrative being presented isn't true. I'm confident most of the parts of this frequently recounted story are quite accurate. These things happened. However, like any big story, there are plenty of smaller tales that get left out, shunted to the sidelines as the meta-narrative makes it mark.

So why am I writing a book on psychedelics? There are surely enough of these in the world right now.

I wanted to tell you some other stories. Some of the stories may be slightly familiar. I'm not trying to create a work of revisionism. Instead, maybe this book will make you question some of the sweeping statements you have likely heard over the past few years, repeated uncritically so often that they're now simply taken as fact.

How about this one: Richard Nixon cracked down on psychedelics in 1970.[4] That was the reason all research suddenly stopped, until some intrepid academics in the early 2000s started things up again with a small study into psilocybin, the main psychoactive molecule in magic mushrooms.[5]

Not exactly true. As we'll learn, most psychedelic research in the United States stopped years before Nixon went all 'war on drugs' in 1970, primarily due to massive shifts in scientific research standards. Plus, not all psychedelic work actually stopped. In some places – like Melbourne, Australia – psychedelic medicine continued up until the mid-1970s. And even when it stopped, it didn't *really* stop. The emergence of MDMA kept both the clinical therapists and those consciousness explorers (known as psychonauts) happy until the mid-1980s; then, just a few years later, a wild psychedelic clinical experiment took place long before the psilocybin breakthrough at the turn of the millennium.

Other stories I want to tell will touch on unusual details that aren't often included in the rush to simplify and condense the modern psychedelic narrative of the last 70 years. Did you know, for example, that infamous beat generation writer William S Burroughs played a major role in discovering the active psychedelic molecule in the ceremonial Amazonian brew ayahuasca? I'm sure you may have heard the tale of a man named Gordon Wasson, who introduced magic mushrooms to the United States in the 1950s, but did you know his landmark anthropological mission to gather samples of the mushrooms was secretly funded by the CIA, and he was accompanied on the journey by an undercover CIA agent who was hunting for new mind-control drugs?

Did you know there are more psychoactive compounds in magic mushrooms beyond the commonly talked about psilocybin? And there is a mysterious paralytic phenomenon striking some magic-mushroom eaters that remains completely unexplained to this day? How about microdosing? I hear so much about that it must be a real thing, right?

Other than recentering the stories we tell about psychedelics, another goal with this book is to position Australia in the global psychedelic renaissance tale. Despite facing a defiantly bleak stretch of several decades during which studying psychedelics was a death knell for your career, Australia has occupied a strangely central position in psychedelic science over the past 70 years.

Melbourne, for example, was one of the few places in the world to continue legally administering psychedelic medicine into the 1970s. It also was one of the first places in the world to restart legal use of psychedelic medicines in 2024. Last out, first in.

EVANGELICAL STORIES ABOUT PSYCHEDELICS HAVE become pervasive, particularly in the hyperbolic early days of the 21st-century renaissance. Psychedelics have suddenly become miracle drugs – cure-alls for whatever ails you. Step right up and enjoy the marvellous medicine of LSD. It will 'change your mind', eliminate depression, cure addiction, rectify eating disorders, fix migraines, heal dementia, reverse aging. You don't even have to take a large dose for it to work. Name a condition and we can likely find someone linking its cure with a psychedelic.

Disentangling the science from the enthusiastic advocacy is difficult but not impossible. Research into what these drugs are doing to our bodies and minds has blown up over the last few years. Academic institutions all over the world are staking a claim in different psychedelic niches.

This wave of new science has heralded fascinating insights into how drugs affect our brain. We are learning how the consumption of certain chemicals can fundamentally alter our perception of the world around us. And we are discovering how chemicals mediate our relationships with others. The story of psychedelic science is nothing less than a story about how we connect with others, form communal bonds and even perceive reality itself.

But first, before we tell that story, we need to do a bit of housekeeping and unpack exactly what we are talking about when we talk about 'psychedelics'.

The word 'psychedelic' wasn't coined until 1956, when psychiatrist Humphry Osmond responded to a letter from writer Aldous Huxley. The pair were corresponding about mescaline and LSD, discussing the drugs and trying to find a label for these novel substances. Huxley introduced the term 'phanerothyme', blending the Greek words *phane* (to appear) and *thymos* (describing the human spirit or soul).

'To make this mundane world sublime, take half a gram of phanerothyme,' Huxley wrote.

Osmond countered with his own pithy rhyme: 'To fathom Hell or soar angelic, just take a pinch of psychedelic.' He was blending the Greek words *psyche* (meaning 'soul', but also more commonly 'mind') and *deloun* (to manifest), and took a bit of poetic licence in changing the spelling and pronunciation to make his phrase rhyme.[6]

As a branding exercise, Osmond's name was perfect. The word took off in the late 1950s, becoming a descriptive badge not only for a type of hallucinogenic drug but also an entire cultural movement. 'Psychedelic' became both a noun and an adjective – or, more strictly for the grammar nerds feeling fury, it became a nominalised adjective.

For Albert Hofmann, in the early 1940s, the word didn't exist. In fact, he initially described LSD as merely an 'amphetamine-type stimulant'.[7] It wasn't until 1947 that the drug was described any differently. Werner Stoll, the son of a colleague working with Hofmann, tried some LSD and used the term 'phantasticum' to describe it. 'Phantasticum' is a wonderful word coined by pharmacologist Louis Lewin in the 1920s. Lewin, whose work focused on uses of the drug mescaline by indigenous peoples of Central America and Mexico, used the word to describe plants that generate hallucinations when consumed by humans.

Unfortunately, 'phantasticum' didn't really stick, and by the early 1960s 'psychedelic' was the word most were using. The category quickly expanded to cover an assortment of psychoactive drugs beyond merely LSD, including psilocybin, mescaline and

DMT. By the 1970s, neuroscientists had discovered the key family of receptors in our brain that seemed to mediate a psychedelic experience. Scientists revealed a common mode of action is shared by these disparate drugs: they all stimulate 5-HT2A serotonin receptors in the brain. And this pharmacological mechanism was subsequently used to group a handful of drugs under a banner we now refer to as 'classic psychedelics'.

LSD, psilocybin, mescaline and DMT all serve as 5-HT2A agonists. These are what we call the classic psychedelics. Of course, as we'll soon learn, the way these drugs work is infinitely more complicated than just simply tickling a single type of receptor in the brain. But also complicating matters is the sheer variety of other drugs often included under the umbrella of 'psychedelics'.

MDMA (ecstasy), ketamine, ibogaine and even cannabis are often grouped under this generalised banner of 'psychedelic science'. Yet all those drugs work on our brain and bodies in very different, and novel, ways. Perhaps a defining characteristic they all share is a renewed scientific focus on their potential therapeutic uses after being classified as illicit psychoactive drugs for so many decades. But are they 'psychedelic' in any subjective sense? And what even is 'psychedelic' in the subjective sense? I'll leave this as an ongoing argument for pharmacologists and psychonauts. And believe me, it *is* an ongoing argument!

FOR OUR PURPOSES, IN THIS BOOK, THE FOCUS IS primarily on three of the four main classic psychedelics, plus a small but important detour into the world of MDMA therapy. Mescaline has strangely been left out of the current wave of new psychedelic research. Not necessarily because it doesn't have therapeutic effects – it likely does – but rather its onerous duration (up to 12 hours) and its strong links to indigenous Native American spiritual use have led most scientists to focus on the other psychedelics. In general, most modern references to 'psychedelic medicine' refer to the classic psychedelics plus MDMA.

In our opening chapter I'll recount the origin story of psychedelic medicine in Australia. This is a story that runs in parallel to the grand American narrative but it offers, perhaps, cautionary lessons for modern psychedelic medicine. Unlike the story in the United States, psychedelic medicine didn't stop in Australia in the mid-1960s. Things kept going in Australia for another decade, and more than a dozen authorised psychiatrists continued to administer the drugs to thousands of patients with almost no governmental oversight. At the same time, bubbling under the surface of psychedelic medicine was a scandal involving a cult using LSD to brainwash its subjects.

I'll also tell the story of Australia's psychedelic research renaissance, or at least its stifled renaissance. It's a frustrating tale of researchers impeded by conservatism until one ambitious clinician finally turned everything on.

The second chapter investigates a rare phenomenon called wood-lover paralysis. For decades strange stories of magic-mushroom paralysis have been shared among psychonauts, but has this been a real phenomenon? Only recently has it been affirmed that yes, it is a real thing. To understand what may be happening, we travel back 65 million years to understand why mushrooms evolved to produce psychedelic molecules.

In learning how some species of mushrooms make psychedelic molecules, we discover that sometimes different kinds of molecules are produced. Wood-lover paralysis is the clue that this is happening, but the knowledge some scientists are now uncovering takes us right up to the cutting edge of genetics and mycology (the science of fungi). This story ultimately points us towards a future world of designer magic mushrooms, custom-engineered for all occasions.

Then I take a look at the very modern phenomenon of psychedelic microdosing. I'm sure you've heard of it. The idea is you can take tiny doses of psychedelics and get boosts of energy, creativity and positive mood. The thing is, no one has really tested whether microdosing is real or not. So I spent some time at Macquarie University in Sydney, where the world's biggest microdosing clinical trial is underway, to find out what we know, what we don't know and how close we are to getting some real answers.

The next chapter takes a dive into the pharmacology of psychedelics. Through the prism of a unique psychedelic molecule called DMT, I look at whether the length of a 'trip' has an effect on its clinical effectiveness. Also, what if we could remove the 'trip' altogether, and are just left with the antidepressant qualities of psychedelics?

The second-last chapter shifts our perspective from the drug side of psychedelic medicine to the psychotherapy side. Here, I talk to some clinicians in Australia who have started delivering these treatments to patients in the real world, using MDMA in particular. What actually happens during the psychotherapy that accompanies psychedelic medicine?

Most of all, I am wondering if we are doing psychedelic medicine the wrong way.

And that's where we'll end up in the final chapter as I try to square my own personal experiences in our modern mental healthcare system with the new hype/hope of psychedelic medicine. How can these powerful drugs fit into our current healthcare models?

Is what we are doing with these drugs in the 21st century really part of an ancient tradition of plant medicine use by cultures all over the world? Or have we concocted a narrow story that helps us pull certain drugs out of illicit framings and into a more acceptable medical container?

I want to set aside the evangelical hype seen in most writing about the psychedelic renaissance. Instead, I want to understand exactly how psychedelics work, and ask how we could be using them outside of the traditional clinical model.

1

HISTORY

PSYCHEDELIC MEDICINE IN AUSTRALIA AND ITS RENAISSANCE

'What they did was not illegal, but highly unethical. We knew, but we couldn't do anything about it.'

Victorian government medical officer John Rutter on the use of psychedelics by some psychiatrists in Melbourne in the 1960s, in 'The Family and its Use of Drugs', *The Age*, 10 September 1990

EVELYN HARRISON WAS 26 YEARS OLD WHEN SHE gave birth to her first and only child at Melbourne's Alfred Hospital in 1958. She named her beautiful daughter Kim but something inside Evelyn didn't feel quite right. Kim was healthy and happy; Evelyn loved her daughter dearly but couldn't shake a strange, inexplicable weight of sadness.

Looking back now, Evelyn understands she was suffering from severe postnatal depression, but back then there was no name for what she was experiencing. By the early 1960s, she was still anguished by feelings of disconnection. During a regular visit to her GP, a new kind of drug treatment was suggested. Little was explained but her doctor asked if she was happy to consent to trying something experimental.

'And I said yes,' Evelyn explained in a 2023 interview with psychedelic historian Jonathan Carmichael, 'because I didn't want to go on feeling depressed about this and I wanted to know why I was depressed.'[1]

Evelyn was referred to a psychiatrist named William Russell Richards. Dr Richards was among a small group of young psychiatrists in Melbourne exploring the therapeutic potential of a new kind of mind-altering medicine known as psychedelics.

The first session took place at a private psychiatric hospital called Newhaven, in the affluent and leafy inner-city suburb of Kew. From the outside, Newhaven looked like a Gothic mansion but, once inside, Evelyn noticed all the trappings of a hospital. She was directed to a private room and given an injection of what she now knows was the psychedelic drug psilocybin.

The drug sessions, which Evelyn participated in about once a month, were mostly undirected. Dr Richards usually sat for a moment with Evelyn while she got settled, then left the room when the 'journey' started. According to Evelyn, the whole idea of the treatment was to 'go deep into yourself' and then tell the doctors what feelings emerged. One of the few times Evelyn was explicitly pushed in a certain direction during a trip was that very first day.

'The first time, I just had hallucinations, and I saw beautiful Christmas trees. Absolutely gorgeous. And they were all in vivid colour. Dr Richards came in and said, "What are you seeing?" And I told him. He said, "Well, that's not going to get you better, is it?" And they just vanished,' Evelyn remembers with a laugh.

After a couple of hours, Evelyn was then directed from her private room into a common area. There she joined a group of about ten patients, all emerging out of their own personal psychedelic trips. For the next few hours, the group shared their experiences, ate some lunch together, and then went home.

This was 1964, and Evelyn continued to participate in these sessions, with the same group, for the next eight years.

'ABSOLUTELY A-BUZZ WITH LSD'

The path to psychedelic medicine in Australia began with a psychiatrist based in the United Kingdom named Ronald Sandison. In the early 1950s, Swiss pharmaceutical company Sandoz began heavily promoting LSD to clinicians around the world. Inside the company, researchers were sure the drug could be useful for some kind of mental health treatment but they weren't exactly sure for what. So they started pushing the drug to psychiatrists for free in the hopes that someone would figure out a clinical use.

In 1952 Sandison went on a research trip to Switzerland. He toured local psychiatric hospitals and, most importantly, visited the labs of Sandoz in Basel. Sandison described the chemists at the Sandoz lab at the time as 'absolutely a-buzz with LSD'.[2] He met up with LSD pioneer Albert Hofmann and returned to the UK with a box of 100 doses of the psychedelic drug.

Upon his return Sandison quickly got to work testing out this new drug on a variety of different patients. By early 1954, he had collected all his preliminary work into a study titled 'The Therapeutic Value of Lysergic Acid Diethylamide in Mental Illness'.[3] The paper proved to be profoundly influential, establishing the foundational framework for a novel kind of LSD psychotherapy that subsequently dominated psychiatric circles in the UK, Europe and Australia for the next two decades.

At the same time, in Melbourne, a young ambitious doctor named Howard Whitaker had recently gained his psychiatric qualifications and was working with the Royal Australian Air Force trying to help veterans who were psychologically scarred from their experiences at war. Whitaker read Sandison's landmark paper and set out to begin the first experiments with psychedelic medicine in Australia.

His work started in 1956 at Newhaven. It's unclear exactly how many patients he treated with LSD over those first few years, but by the early 1960s he decided to complete a more rigorous investigation into the usefulness of the drug. In hindsight, Whitaker openly referred to his early tests with LSD as unsuccessful. In a paper published in 1964, he suggested his initial attempts failed because he believed 'the psychotherapy then used was inadequate'.[4]

Between 1961 and 1964 Whitaker treated 100 patients with LSD, based on a protocol closely resembling that described by Sandison in the UK. This paradigm of LSD treatment in Australia stood apart from what was emerging in North America; there were two schools of drug-assisted psychotherapy being practised at the time and they couldn't have been more dramatically different.[5]

In North America the dominant treatment modality in the 1960s involved extremely high doses of either LSD or psilocybin (at least 250 micrograms of LSD, or 25 milligrams of psilocybin).[6]

The goal was to engender transformational insights in a patient by giving them what has been called a 'mystical experience'. Patients usually only undertook a small handful of drug sessions, and the goal was to generate an experience of awe and connectedness that seemed to correlate with improvements in mental health.

The alternative method, practised by Whitaker and his European counterparts, was known as psycholytic therapy.[7] Here, the psychiatrist uses lower doses of the drug, more frequently, as a crucial adjunct to psychotherapy. These lower doses (spanning anywhere from 30 to 150 micrograms for LSD and 3 to 15 milligrams for psilocybin)[8] were not intended to generate a completely dissociated state but instead were used to trigger what Whitaker called a 'revivification of early trauma'.[9]

Whitaker's core hypothesis, echoed by Sandison and other psycholytic therapy practitioners, was that 'the essence of neurosis and personality disorder is the distortion of adult adjustment by the persistence of patterns of emotional reaction from infancy'.[10] This distinctly Freudian framing for psychoanalysis suggested psychedelic drugs were effective at recovering repressed childhood memories – a framework that is still to this day consistently applied to psychedelics.

As Sandison laid out in his 1954 paper, this kind of therapy is not a short-term intervention. Instead, he recommended each patient endure at least half a dozen drug sessions over several weeks to try to delve deep into their repressed mind.

The results of Whitaker's work, described across two papers published in 1964,[11] revealed this kind of LSD psycholytic therapy to be very hit-and-miss. He described 47 cases as 'successfully' treated by the therapy, 18 cases as 'borderline', and 35 cases that simply failed to respond at all.

By the mid-1960s, psychedelic medicine was widespread in Australia. With no formal patient records or registry tracking, it's hard to quantify exactly how many psychiatrists were working with psychedelics. It's likely several dozen across the country were administering the drugs, and psychiatric hospitals such as Newhaven in Melbourne became significant psychedelic treatment hubs.

'IT WAS A MIXED GROUP'

Evelyn's psychedelic therapy group was one of Dr Richards' first at Newhaven; kicking off in 1964, it included about as diverse a bunch of people as you could get.

> There was a paedophile who'd been handed over by the police to be there. He had to go. We had concentration camp victims. We had bipolar people. We had two homosexuals, male and female. And a couple of other people who were dealing with alcohol and smoking.
>
> So it was a mixed group. They were a fairly intelligent group of people and some of them came from quite well-known families.

Over the next few years, Evelyn saw lots more psychedelic therapy groups form around her. By the end of the decade, her sister, brother-in-law and several friends had all had a run at some psychedelic therapy. Each had been part of a unique group of people.

From Evelyn's perspective the group aspect of the treatment was crucial to its beneficial outcomes and she found it deeply valuable. Everyone supported each other as they delved into some of the most traumatic parts of their lives. Occasional one-on-one sessions between Dr Richards and his patients helped facilitate the direction things were going, but the entire process was fundamentally geared at a kind of self-work.

'Dr Richards would comment on certain things, but he wouldn't tell you what to do. You had to do it yourself. It was definitely a self-help thing. And it was very tough because some of the things that came up were very painful, and they'd be put away, and you never wanted to look at them again. It's like crawling over broken glass, but we did, and it really did help.'

After about a year of sessions at Newhaven, Evelyn began to sense something was a little off. She considered herself an empathic person, and the psychedelics seemed to amplify this sense. One day she approached Dr Richards with a wild assertion: the matron of the hospital was a Nazi.

Evelyn's instinct turned out to be correct. A scandal was brewing in Melbourne psychiatric circles. A cult had infiltrated the Newhaven hospital. The matron, and Dr Howard Whitaker, had fallen under the influence of a group known as 'The Family'.

A week after Evelyn raised her concern with Dr Richards, the group moved out of Newhaven. From then, up until 1972, the group's sessions took place at a space in Richmond, adjacent to the Epworth Hospital.

Evelyn described her therapeutic process as slow and difficult. Psychedelics were no quick fix for her. Instead, they gradually allowed her to see, and work through, trauma from her childhood that had been deeply suppressed. One of the key moments in her treatment came when Dr Richards identified a point in Evelyn's life that she was holding onto so tightly it couldn't be unlocked. One drug session stepped things up and Evelyn was given a very high intravenous dose of psilocybin. The trip came on fast, and the memories soon followed.

> I remembered I was seven years old. I was wearing a little velvet dress with a lace collar. We were in the botanical gardens in Melbourne, my mother and father, walking through the gardens, and I was just playing around and

> there was an old stone building at the side, and I ran around it and there was a man there. And he exposed himself and put my hand on his penis.
>
> He said, 'If you tell your parents, I'll kill you.' I ran back to my parents and I was too scared to say anything. But for years, when I was happy, I'd think, 'Oh, something awful is gonna happen.' And I couldn't understand why I always felt this.
>
> When I went back to that incident and saw what had happened, that feeling went away completely. I no longer had any fear of things going wrong for me. That's how it worked. It took you to look, with an adult brain, at what a child was seeing.

For Evelyn the psychedelic treatment had unlocked a repressed memory. The childhood trauma that emerged was new to her but it helped her understand and work through a feeling of anxiety that permeated her everyday life as an adult. The treatment was working exactly as it should, but, as we'll learn, the revelation of forgotten childhood trauma under the influence of psychedelics isn't a positive experience for everyone.

THE VICTORIAN EXCEPTION

Nixon, hippies, Timothy Leary and counterculture's threat to the status quo. These are the general points hit by most stories telling the tale of why psychedelic medicine hit a wall and stopped in the 1960s. Recreational use of LSD had dragged psychedelics out of the offices of psychiatrists and into youth culture. Researchers leapt out of their academic shackles, becoming proselytisers of psychedelics. Leary in particular turned into a key counterculture figure after being fired from his job as a psychology lecturer at

Harvard University in 1963. His studies had rapidly turned into ethical quagmires as he began regularly consuming psychedelics with his students.

This mashing up of psychedelic research with countercultural enlightenment turned the whole project of psychedelic science upside down. Several US states quickly banned LSD, California being one of the first in 1966, before Nixon finally got serious blanket prohibitions sorted by the end of the decade.

It is certainly true that these social factors played a role in the growing wave of panicked media reports about LSD, but this wasn't the real reason psychedelic medicine ended up slowing down in the 1960s. The real reason was our threshold for scientific proof changed and psychedelic practitioners struggled to keep up.

Historian Matthew Oram spent years digging through US Food and Drug Administration files on LSD research from the 1960s and he discovered something surprising.[12] He saw a government regulatory agency that was actually working to keep psychedelic medicine and research alive. In the files he found little evidence of any attempt to stop the research. What really hampered psychedelic science and medicine in the 1960s was the passing of a new law known as the Kefauver–Harris Amendment.

In the late 1950s, one of the biggest disasters in modern medical history took place. More than 10 000 children were born with severe physical deformities after their mothers took a drug called thalidomide during their pregnancies. Thousands of other pregnancies ended in miscarriage. The drug first appeared in 1957, and was marketed as a cure-all for everything from anxiety to insomnia, but in particular it was used during pregnancy to treat morning sickness.[13] However, it had never been tested on pregnant people because there were no clear regulations on determining efficacy for drugs.

The thalidomide scandal reverberated around the world across the early 1960s and the result was new attitudes towards testing the safety and efficacy of medicines. One of the first big legal changes came in the US with the Kefauver–Harris Amendment. This law required clear clinical proof of efficacy and safety before a drug was legally allowed to be marketed. Clinical trials subsequently became more controlled and more rigorous, and this ultimately led to safer and more efficacious medicines.

But for psychedelics this was the beginning of the end. As Oram elegantly argues in his book *The Trials of Psychedelic Therapy,* early researchers had always struggled to prove psychedelics were effective medicines. They certainly worked for some people, but they also didn't work for just as many. And once empirical research standards were introduced, psychedelics seemed ill-suited for these methods of evaluation.

ALONGSIDE THESE EVOLVING MEASURES OF RESEARCH efficacy, psychedelics were taking a big PR hit in the news, with increasing numbers of 'bad trips' being reported leading to medical emergencies. This prompted Swiss manufacturer Sandoz to reconsider its general practice of sending free psychedelics to those researchers who asked. Most current narratives date the formal end of psychedelic medicine to early 1966, when Sandoz allegedly made the worldwide decision to withdraw LSD, psilocybin and all related substances from distribution.

The popular story goes that Sandoz was spooked by the increasingly broad recreational uses of their drugs. Governments around the world were cracking down on psychedelics, and in the United States, figures like Timothy Leary, Ralph Metzner and Richard Alpert (aka Ram Dass) were creating a funnel between clinical psychedelic work and recreational use. So Sandoz pulled the pin and said, 'No more.' As reported by outlets including *The New York Times* and *Rolling Stone,* and reiterated by writers such as Michael Pollan and researchers like Robin Carhart-Harris,

Sandoz apparently completely stopped manufacturing these drugs.[14] The good times were over.

But that story turned out to be not *entirely* true. While Sandoz did indeed dramatically withdraw its psychedelic substances from international distribution in 1966, it didn't stop manufacturing the drugs. And alongside the global withdrawal were some significant caveats that meant the story played out a little differently in countries like Australia.

Ian Collins, Sandoz's Australian representative, sent a letter to doctors and health departments around the country on 12 May 1966.[15] The letter indicated supply of its drugs in Australia was of no immediate concern to the company. However, he noted the 'serious deterioration in the situation overseas, where the misuse of hallucinogenic drugs has reached dangerous proportions in certain countries'.

Collins explained Sandoz would 'no longer bear the responsibility for the further allocation and distribution of these substances'. But there were exceptions that could be made in situations 'where the government authorities are willing to undertake complete responsibility for the allocation and distribution of these materials'.

Essentially, Sandoz was content to continue supplying psychedelics to those who wanted them but was not going to take any responsibility for their distribution; that needed to be up to the government. In the United States this exception was not considered, even for a moment. Between the noise of counterculture and the government's itch for prohibition, psychedelic drugs were swiftly banned, and by 1967 almost every research program in the country had been shut down.

A similar story played out in the United Kingdom. No government agency wanted to go near psychedelics, so the Sandoz withdrawal slowly shuttered every clinical and research program in the region.

However, things weren't the same over in Australia. A psychedelic counterculture was certainly materialising, but it seemed to exist in a world completely apart from that of the medical profession. No researcher or psychiatrist had taken up the role of an Aussie Tim Leary crossing the streams between medical and recreational uses of psychedelics. Instead, there was a small group of doctors who had been quietly working with the drugs.

In Victoria a handful of psychiatrists soon began pressuring the state's Department of Health. Howard Whitaker led the charge, pressing Victoria's Chief Health Officer to take control of these drugs in a way that would satisfy Sandoz's requirements for governmental oversight. By June 1966 a state scheduling subcommittee had agreed the drugs could be 'valuable and useful' in a clinical context.[16] So regulations were recommended that allowed psychedelics to be administered by authorised psychiatrists under controlled conditions.

A special committee was appointed by the Victorian health department, delegated to draft a system by which LSD and psilocybin could be possessed and used by certain permitted clinicians. Howard Whitaker took a prominent position on this committee, and by the end of 1966 the state had enacted a novel set of regulations, making it one of the few places in the world to legally continue the practice of psychedelic medicine.

The next year Sandoz was presented with the new Victorian Department of Health regulations. The state's Chief Health Officer was to take possession of the drugs and distribute them to psychiatrists who completed the necessary applications. Sandoz was satisfied. In early March 1967, the first legal delivery of state-controlled LSD and psilocybin arrived at the offices of the Department of Health in Melbourne – stamped with the Sandoz brand, and ready for distribution to a small network of authorised Melbourne-based psychiatrists.

'YOUR HUSBAND IS A PSYCHOPATH'

'I don't think the drugs were any help at all. I don't think I should have been given them. I thought they were given to psychiatric patients. I wasn't a psychiatric patient. I was a nice, lovely country girl with a cheerful personality who was married to a lunatic.'

It was 1968 and Vivien Achia was 23 years old, with a healthy baby daughter, Alice, and a charismatic husband named Jack. Six months into their marriage, Vivien was deeply unsettled. Her 'happily ever after' story had not come to pass. Instead, her husband was never around and Vivien became convinced it was because something was wrong with her.

Friends recommended she seek marriage counselling and that's how Vivien ended up meeting a psychiatrist named John Mackay at Newhaven hospital.

> I said, 'My husband's never home. Is there something wrong with me?' And [Mackay's] response to that was, 'We can quickly get into your subconscious and see what's driving you if we give you some LSD.' He said that will cut out two or three years of talk, two or three years of counselling. I was scared of drugs. But I thought, 'Well, if it makes a difference, I'll do it.'

For the next few months, Vivien engaged in a form of psychedelic therapy practised by the team at Newhaven. Her husband would drop her off at the hospital on a Saturday morning. She would be taken upstairs and ushered into a private room. A nurse would give her an injection of LSD and cover her eyes with a silk scarf, and they would sit together quietly while the drug did its work.

Occasionally the nurse would help direct or interpret Vivien's hallucinations, and by the evening a sedative would be administered to end the trip. Vivien would stay overnight at the hospital, writing her reflections on the experience in a journal the next morning before her husband arrived to take her home.

Two weeks after a drug session, Vivien would meet up with John Mackay to discuss her experiences, and then two weeks later she would have another LSD session at the hospital.

Every drug session was different. Initially Vivien felt happy and relaxed, but as time passed she began to get anxious and afraid. Her trips were increasingly filled with images of dragons and demonic nurses. Nothing was being learned, and Vivien was feeling more traumatised as the months progressed.

By her sixth LSD treatment, things had reached a breaking point. During a particularly intense session, a supposedly repressed memory emerged from Vivien's subconscious. The nurse accompanying her during the session assured her this was a real memory that Vivien had been suppressing all these years. She was told coming to terms with it would help her overcome her mental health struggles. But Vivien was not convinced. She was certain the events being recalled could not have happened and became deeply uncomfortable with the whole process.

> And that's where I came up with my concern about not being able to distinguish [reality] from fantasy once the genie's out of the bottle. Once you give someone LSD and you scramble up their memories and their wishes and fantasies, false memories are a very real risk, because you can no longer distinguish what's real and what's not.

Although Vivien's story with LSD ended there, her experiences with John Mackay and Newhaven didn't. Mackay grew interested in Vivien's husband Jack and invited him to Newhaven to have an LSD treatment. Jack eagerly agreed, seemingly enjoying the experience so much that he skipped out of the hospital overnight and went fishing.

Visiting Mackay for the last time, Vivien was told she was healthy. Mackay said there was nothing wrong with her, but then added, 'Your husband ... he's a psychopath and we want him to come in for full-time psychiatric treatment.'

Looking back, Vivien's only positive takeaway from the whole experience was learning she wasn't the problem but that in fact it was her husband with the psychiatric issues. She is convinced that with the aid of a perceptive psychologist, she could have reached this conclusion without going through months of LSD experiences.

The marriage, of course, didn't last very long. Jack's erratic behaviour led him to disappear to Queensland, while Vivien, years later, met another man and lived a long, happy and eventful life.

Her memories of Newhaven and Mackay are not particularly fond ones, but she doesn't feel ill will towards those who worked at the hospital. To her at least, Mackay and the nurses at Newhaven were sincere in their attempts to use this novel treatment to help.

But Vivien may have been one of the lucky ones, as things behind the scenes at Newhaven during the late 1960s were rapidly becoming darker and more nefarious.

INITIATIONS, THE CULT AND A 'FUCKING WITCH'

In 1964, Howard Whitaker was introduced to a woman named Anne Hamilton.[17] Personally, at the time, Whitaker admitted he was 'mixed up in his religious beliefs'.[18] After several years of administering LSD and psilocybin to patients, he had finally taken the advice laid out on Sandoz's label for LSD and tried the drug himself.

Anne Hamilton was in her early forties, a yoga teacher and a budding guru. A colleague of Whitaker's, Raynor Johnson, had already fallen under the influence of Hamilton, as she deployed psychedelic drugs as strategic weapons of persuasion. Johnson had been 'initiated' by Hamilton the previous year, in a ceremony thought to have involved magic mushrooms.

In Whitaker, Johnson spotted an opportunity. Whitaker was a man in crisis with a strong connection to psychedelic medicine. Johnson had long thought a spiritual element was missing in clinical LSD-assisted psychotherapy, so what better moment to connect a clinical practitioner with someone he believed was a spiritual teacher?

That first meeting between Whitaker and Hamilton took place at Raynor Johnson's home. The significant event was richly described in *The Family*, a well-researched book by Chris Johnston and Rosie Jones on what would ultimately become one of Australia's most notorious cults. Hamilton and Whitaker talked about religion: 'She told him she could see auras and the future, spiritually heal those in need, and commune with the paranormal. He returned and saw her around ten times, and then she told him he should try and enter her spiritual realm.' Whitaker later said he was 'quite impressed' with Hamilton's knowledge: 'I was reading up about the things she was on about … Christianity, Hindu religions, Muslim religions, and I checked up on different things she said.'[19]

At some point in 1964, Whitaker himself was 'initiated' by Hamilton. Again, at Johnson's house, in a ceremony that likely involved the consumption of some kind of psychedelic drug, Whitaker promised his allegiance and obedience to Hamilton, the Spiritual Teacher. 'Anne said because of her status as a guru she was able to take over responsibility for resolving our karma … and that's how we took steps on the path towards ultimate liberation,' Whitaker later recounted.[20]

Hamilton stressed the importance of loyalty and the severity of the ultimate crime of betrayal by citing a mantra, which Whitaker was told was so secret it couldn't even be written down. 'The oath and obedience and secrecy is repeated over and over,' he later explained. 'That's the hold Anne has on people. After May 1964, quite quickly Anne started to tell me what to do with my life.'[21]

From that point forward, Hamilton became a frequent presence at Newhaven hospital. She wasn't a nurse, but she used the space to run yoga and meditation classes, gradually exerting her influence over staff and patients. The head matron of the hospital, Joan Vilimek, soon became another initiate of Hamilton's and things went downhill fast.

The hospital was both a site of recruitment and indoctrination for Hamilton's burgeoning cult. John Mackay and the other resident psychiatrist, Harry Bethune, began serving Hamilton's wishes. Members of Hamilton's cult would be admitted under false names and given high doses of LSD or psilocybin while Hamilton and other group members performed what they called 'clearings'. Ronald Sandison first coined the term 'clearing' to describe the process of a therapeutic LSD experience. Here, Whitaker and the cult appropriated it into a term to describe the regular brainwashing designed to keep members under Hamilton's spell.

Separately, hospital patients were also seen as potential new recruits for the group. Several instances have been recounted where a hospital patient, alone in a room under the influence of psychedelics, would suddenly come face to face with a woman in a billowing white dress. This woman claimed she was Jesus Christ and the solution to all their problems.

Some patients succumbed, joining Anne's growing flock. Others, like Toby Zoates, saw through the insane charade and got out of the hospital quick smart. Zoates had been admitted by John Mackay in 1969 after another cult member eyed him for recruitment. Zoates was gay and had been convinced his homosexuality was a mental illness. Mackay told him ten sessions of LSD therapy spread across three months should serve as an effective 'psychic clearing'.[22]

After three sessions it was clear Zoates wasn't responding well to the treatment, at least insofar as he wasn't becoming the sycophantic spiritual follower they were trying to mould. So in the fourth session they introduced Anne Hamilton, after Mackay had primed Zoates with a second booster shot of LSD:

> [Hamilton] sat by my bed and tried to mesmerize me with admonishments to vomit it all up, all the times I'd been raped, tortured, murdered, and in turn all the murders I'd committed, the blood-letting, the disembowelling, in all my past lives, and I retched for her benefit, my body became twisted and misshapen, but I still didn't become the pliable fool. I actually thought, 'Who is this fucking witch? What a freak, she'd scare the bejesus out of the Devil!' Finally she gave up on me, leaving me to be molded into her clay Golem another day, probably towards the end of the ten psycho sessions I was booked in for.[23]

Early the next morning, as the sun was coming up, Zoates quietly snuck out of the hospital, running through the garden and jumping over the back fence. He never returned to Newhaven.

'Fuck having ten sessions of that nonsense,' he wrote, years later.

WHEN THE FIRST LEGAL DELIVERIES OF LSD AND psilocybin arrived at the Victorian Department of Health in

1967, following the establishment of the state's new regulatory framework, there were 19 psychiatrists in Melbourne authorised to hold and administer these psychedelic drugs.[24] Of those 19, five were affiliated in some way with Newhaven psychiatric hospital. And three – Howard Whitaker, John Mackay and Harry Bethune – were explicitly under direction from Anne Hamilton, their Spiritual Teacher.

After applying to use psychedelic drugs, the only legal requirement for psychiatrists in Victoria was keeping a detailed register of how many doses of drugs they were holding and when they were administered. There was no other oversight tracking how the drugs were used, what they were used for, or even if they were working as effective medicines.

The first, and only, compliance inspection checking in on each of the authorised psychiatrists took place in mid-1969, a full two years after legal deliveries had kicked off. In a report that was uncovered by historian Megan Lomax in 2017, it was revealed that only one of the 19 authorised psychiatrists had their regulatory compliance deemed 'excellent'. A few others were deemed 'fair' but a remarkable 15 practitioners had both their record-keeping and storage practices classified as 'unsatisfactory'.[25]

Most of these non-compliance issues centred on vague documentation. Some records were completely out of date, while others were loosely gathered on scraps of paper. Where doses ended up was frequently unclear. Insecure drug storage problems abounded: the inspectors found some psychedelic stocks randomly stored in unlocked cupboards among office stationery.

Howard Whitaker, one of the members of the committee responsible for drafting the regulations in the first place, was ironically found to be the most non-compliant of all authorised prescribers. The report described his records as 'chaotic' and noted inaccuracies in his balances of drug stocks. According to the inspectors, the cupboard in his desk containing the drugs had only just been fitted with what looked like a new lock.

What happened following this stark report?

Absolutely nothing.

In July 1969 Victoria's Chief Health Officer issued a stern letter to all authorised psychiatrists. The letter reminded them of their legal obligations to keep a detailed register and have secure storage facilities. And that was that. No further inspections were conducted for compliance between this moment in 1969 and the ultimate broad ban on all uses of LSD and psilocybin in Australia by 1975.

The Newhaven scandal didn't emerge into the public consciousness until the 1980s. At the time, however, it seems the inappropriate use of psychedelic drugs by some psychiatrists was common knowledge among both government officials and other psychiatrists.

The Victorian Department of Health was allegedly aware of what was going on at Newhaven but had no legal way to stop it. John Rutter, a medical officer from the government's Poisons division, was recruited by the Department of Health to try to find a way to eradicate clinical use of psychedelics, but there was little he could do. Speaking years later, Rutter said what was going on at Newhaven may have been unethical, but it wasn't illegal. There was simply nothing the Department of Health could do to police psychedelic practitioners beyond issuing a $200 fine.[26]

Across the roughly 15-year period in which psychedelic medicine was legally practised in Victoria, it has been estimated that up to 10 000 patients potentially experienced the treatment.[27] Hospitals all over Melbourne were practising psychedelic medicine, including St Vincent's Hospital in Fitzroy and the Epworth in Richmond. No records remain, so we have no idea who these patients were, what they were treated for, and whether their treatments were successful.

As for the Newhaven scandal, Howard Whitaker left the hospital – and Anne Hamilton's cult – suddenly in late 1969. He excommunicated himself from Hamilton, later suggesting he had begun to see her methods as devious and her teachings as 'crap'.[28] He shifted to working in rural hospitals, spending the early 1970s at Beechworth's Mayday Hills Hospital, allegedly still administering LSD and psilocybin therapeutically until its prohibition in 1975.

The cult of Anne Hamilton – later known as Anne Hamilton-Byrne – grew increasingly unhinged over the following years, culminating in a police raid in the late 1980s bringing everything to a crashing halt. Anne passed away in 2019 in a nursing home in the hills outside of Melbourne.

John Mackay is one of the few major players from this era still alive. He lives a reclusive life in the Dandenong Ranges, still believing in both the power of psychedelic medicine and the wisdom of Anne Hamilton-Byrne, his Spiritual Teacher.

'AT FIRST IT KNOCKS YOU AROUND A LITTLE BIT'

Evelyn continued her frequent psilocybin group therapy sessions with William Russell Richards until things abruptly stopped in 1972. It's unclear what exactly prompted the sudden culmination of Dr Richards' Melbourne work but, according to Evelyn, he shut things down relatively quickly and left the country.

How many psilocybin sessions did Evelyn have in the eight years she spent doing the treatment? She doesn't know, but she can say it was 'a damn lot of them'. From her perspective, the treatment was long, hard work – and a crucial part of the process was learning how to 'use' the drugs.

> In the end you have to learn to control it. You have to grab it when it hits you. You have to direct it to where you want to look at, and you learn to do that. You learn to say, 'Now this week I'm going to investigate why I'm doing so and so.' And you have to direct your brain towards it, and it will work.
>
> But it takes a while to get to that. At first, it knocks you around a little bit with the hallucinations. Some of them are a bit frightening, but I'm not frightened of anything now.

Ultimately, Evelyn's psychedelic treatment led to the end of her marriage. It became clear that the relationship was toxic, and by the time the sessions ended in 1972 she felt confident and in control of her life. She later remarried. Today she describes her psychedelic experiences as 'one of the most marvellous things that ever happened'.

In the 50 years since those sessions, Evelyn has not taken any recreational drugs or craved the experience of psilocybin. She knows she is one of the lucky ones. The treatment certainly didn't work for everyone. In fact, there were significant controversies, even in Evelyn's small group. Two participants took their own lives over the course of the treatment, and Evelyn is not at all flippant about how seriously these drugs should be considered. Psychedelic therapy undeniably worked for her but she knows better than anyone that the drugs can be damaging when given to the wrong patients in the wrong contexts.

> The result of this treatment has stabilised my life. I take each day as it comes, conscious of the beauty around me. I count myself so lucky to have been in the right place at the right time ... I am 92 now and have had a very successful, happy marriage for 40 years.

> I am not afraid to die. Psilocybin changed my life for the better. I love this planet, its diversity and stunning beauty. There are secrets to learn, a cosmos to explore, and maybe an exciting hereafter or universal consciousness. One more big mystery ...

THE AUSTRALIAN RENAISSANCE

By 1970, the US federal government had effectively banned all uses of psychedelic drugs. International prohibitions, on the other hand, took a little longer to take hold. It took a couple of years for the United Nations to agree on including psychedelics in its international prohibition, and it wasn't until 1975 that the full block was put into place. Up until then, Sandoz was still supplying psychedelics to the Victorian government but, as soon at the UN put up its firewall, everything stopped.

All research and clinical uses were ended. At least, technically.

Despite a freeze on above-ground research, dedicated psychonauts and citizen scientists all over the world continued vigilantly working with these drugs: learning, listening, experimenting. Those who persevered in the shadows laid the foundations for much of the legal work emerging in the 21st-century renaissance.

All good stories start somewhere, and the first weekend in December 2010 is as good a place as any to situate the beginning of Australia's above-ground psychedelic renaissance. Here, an assortment of psychonauts, drug nerds, botanists, scientists, doctors, chemists, hippies and counterculture freaks infiltrated the hallowed halls of the University of Melbourne to hold a unique kind of conference.

It was a gathering of a group called Entheogenesis Australis (or, more informally to those in the know, EGA). Presentations at the conference looked at the current state of drug law reform in Australia, how cough medicine could be used as a shamanic sacrament and how ayahuasca ceremonies in Australia are taking on a novel cultural context. It was a diverse, weird and altogether stimulating weekend of presentations.

I know because I was there: all day, every day, in the very front row.

I was the 'tech guy' at the conference. I'd been friends with the EGA crew for a few years. In a past life, I was a DJ, involved in organising some outdoor parties, and the Australian bush party scene (or 'doof' community) was an incredible melting pot of alternative subcultures. So the EGA crew frequently crossed my path, and over time I helped out with their events – and they helped out with mine. I even gave my first ever public talk at one of the earliest EGA events in 2006. (The talk was about how outdoor 'doof' parties resemble indigenous community rituals, in both form and function. I found the notes for the talk recently. It's not the most embarrassing thing I wrote at that age, that's for sure.)

Ambling conversations on the side of dancefloors in the Aussie bush stoked my interest in all the odd fringe science that filled the heads of these pioneering psychonauts. Only now, in hindsight, do I realise how this shaggy band of weirdos so significantly shaped Australia's current world of psychedelic science and medicine.

Being the tech guy at the EGA conference in 2010 was a pretty simple job 95 per cent of the time: set up each speaker's PowerPoint presentation and make sure it all runs smoothly. The frantic stress of those moments when a video wouldn't play properly or a microphone dropped out were few in a space as grand as the University of Melbourne. For most of the weekend, I could just sit and get a front-row view of all the presentations.

The headlining speaker at the conference was a researcher from the United States named Rick Doblin. It was Doblin's first visit to Australia and the EGA team bringing him here felt like a bit of a coup – a wild step into the world of respectable international science by some long-haired Aussie psychonauts. Doblin was instrumental in shepherding psychedelic medicine back to the mainstream. His work has primarily focused on MDMA, and it went all the way back to when the drug was first made illegal in the mid-1980s.

In 1986 Doblin founded an organisation called the Multidisciplinary Association for Psychedelic Studies (MAPS). His ostensible goal was to bring MDMA back into the world of psychological medicine after its escape into the party scene brought clinical use to a standstill, in ways distinctly reminiscent of 1960s psychedelic prohibition. (I say 'ostensible goal' because Doblin has been clear his research work is designed to serve as a Trojan Horse for broader drug legalisation. He believes medical use of psychedelics will pave the way for a wave of social acceptability that opens the door to full legalisation. He often talks about a utopia in 2070 where all drugs are legal and accessible via a licensing process similar to the way we regulate driving a car.)

Doblin painstakingly spent years scraping together funding to slowly chip away at the studies necessary to prove MDMA safe to use as a medicine, and by 2010 he was a bit of a counterculture hero. He'd pushed through the science showing MDMA was safe in humans, and then started the clinical work to establish it as a medicine to treat post-traumatic stress disorder.

Across two expansive talks at the EGA conference, Doblin described where his research currently was (he was in the thick of early Phase 2 human trials with MDMA for post-traumatic stress disorder) and where he saw the future of psychedelic medicine. It was a wild and electric moment for the Australian psychedelic community. A sense something really big was happening swept through the auditorium, and the ripples of this wave led to more than just abstract enthusiasm.

The day after the conference concluded, Doblin took part

in a smaller workshop with a group of local researchers. The gathering of around 30 people was kind of like a hyperfocused brainstorming session around one central question: 'What needs to happen to get a clinical psychedelic trial going in Australia?'

The outcome of that day was the founding of an organisation called PRISM – Psychedelic Research in Science and Medicine. Several influential figures in Australia's psychedelic community contributed to the birth of PRISM: Darklight, Tim Payne, Stephen Bright, Steve McDonald, Jonathan Carmichael and Torsten Wiedemann. Dr Martin Williams stepped into the role of president. Williams had a rich background in medicinal chemistry and pharmacology, plus he had worked in the past to help formally establish Entheogenesis Australis as a legally recognised association.

With the backing of a generous financial pledge from Doblin's research organisation MAPS, the group set to work on starting an Australian clinical trial testing MDMA for post-traumatic stress disorder. By the beginning of 2012, the crew were ready to take their first big swing. They had done the work to formally set up PRISM as a charity organisation, and they'd spent months developing a robust clinical trial protocol, mirroring the work MAPS had been doing at other sites around the world. Everything was sorted; a community clinic had been found as a location, and a local psychiatrist with pre-existing MAPS therapist training was brought in to lead the trial. The final hurdle was getting an ethics committee to sign off on the trial, a crucial prerequisite for any clinical research in Australia.

In late February 2012 came D-day for the team. The ethics committee met to discuss the application, they spoke to the lead psychiatrist, and then swiftly said 'No thanks'. It was a crushing result.

The ethics board flagged a number of issues with PRISM's application. They weren't comfortable with the safety implications of this kind of research taking place in a community clinic as opposed to a hospital. They also questioned the impartiality of the research, suggesting a group like PRISM was an 'advocacy organisation'. But above all, Martin Williams feels the lead psychiatrist on this bold first proposal just dropped the ball.

Looking back more than a decade later, Williams is still bruised by the knockback. The path of psychedelic research in Australia would have been fundamentally different if that ethics committee had taken a chance back in 2012.

'In retrospect, it was just way too early for us to be doing any of that,' Williams said to me in 2025, with a resigned shrug. 'We didn't have any research or clinical trial background. So we sort of licked our wounds and said, "Okay, well we better talk to some proper clinical trial people."'

'UNETHICAL AND ILLEGAL'

Take two for the MDMA trial came in 2013. The PRISM team connected with an experienced psychiatrist whose private clinical practice had managed a number of psychiatric trials. This ticked all the boxes that had been lacking in their last attempt.

Things progressed quickly. The old trial protocol was dusted off and it was all systems go. Until it reached the practice's clinical trial manager. This manager straight-up refused to engage in the trial, expressing great discomfort at the notion of working with what they saw as illicit drugs. The 'ecstasy' taboo was strong, and it didn't take much to come up against someone who simply wouldn't be associated with MDMA, that 'dangerous party drug'.

There was no way around this intractable roadblock, and PRISM notched up failure number two.

A couple more years passed, with the team unable to find any organisation or institution in Australia willing to mount a psychedelic clinical trial. And then a psychiatrist named Nigel Strauss entered the scene.

It was 2015 and Strauss was an adjunct professor at Melbourne's Deakin University. He had recently returned from training in the UK to become a MAPS-accredited MDMA therapist. Never one to take things slowly, Strauss swiftly moved things along. He and Martin Williams again polished the old MDMA for PTSD trial protocol, got their ducks in a row, and submitted an application to the university's ethics committee. This was as good as it got: a respectable academic institution and a long-standing psychiatry professor. Surely this one would work?

The night before the proposal was set to be evaluated by the ethics committee, Strauss received a striking telephone call from the university's vice-chancellor. Strauss was told the trial proposal would be blocked by the university. Afraid to damage its reputation, the university claimed it would never be affiliated with MAPS, the American organisation that was helping sponsor the trial.

'MAPS was not considered to be a socially responsible organisation because it engaged in activities that were unethical and illegal,' the formal rejection letter from Deakin University stated.[29]

Somewhat ironically, at virtually the same moment, across the Pacific Ocean in North America, MAPS representatives including Rick Doblin were meeting with the US Food and Drug Administration, presenting Phase 2 trial data and hatching plans for Phase 3 clinical trials. While Australian universities were considering the work unethical and illegal, US regulatory agencies were racing to move things forward into large-scale clinical stages.

BY 2017, THE BURGEONING INTERNATIONAL RENAISsance in psychedelic science and medicine was well and truly cooking. The FDA had given MAPS' work with MDMA for post-traumatic stress disorder its 'Breakthrough Therapy' designation, and Phase 3 human trials were about to kick off. A handful of other psychedelic studies were also brewing around the world, including LSD work in Switzerland and psilocybin investigations in the UK.

Despite a few quiet years in Australia, the EGA community decided to roll the dice one more time and hold a massive outdoor psychedelic symposium. Staged in the gorgeous surrounds of Victoria's Lake Eildon, the event brought together another mind-bendingly disparate collection of people from around Australia, and the world.

Ethnobotanist Kathleen Harrison talked about psychedelic plants and indigenous ritual, while Rick Doblin was again present, this time to show how far his work had progressed since that first visit back in 2010. And an assortment of Australian presenters covered all corners of psychedelic culture – aboveground, underground, and everything in between.

On the Saturday evening, before a parade of international headliners, Martin Williams stepped on stage to give a short presentation titled 'Intro to Psychedelic Research in Australia'.

Williams began with a joke ... sort of.

He was going to talk about the status of psychedelic research in Australia, he told us. Then he flicked to a new slide. It was blank. He thanked the audience for their time and pretended to walk off.

Titters of uncomfortable laughter spread through the crowd. It was a bitter moment. Internationally, psychedelic science was flourishing, but in Australia it was still sitting cross-legged on the fringes of credibility. Despite years of work, PRISM couldn't find any organisation in Australia willing to step up and back serious psychedelic research.

Williams' talk only lasted ten minutes. He expressed hope that things would change soon but, after nearly a decade of personally pushing up against closed doors, it was clear he was tired.

Little did he know that a young clinical psychologist named Marg Ross was in the crowd, listening closely to his presentation. And she was anxious, because she had a decision to make that could change the path of psychedelic medicine in Australia for everyone.

'DEATH AND REBIRTH'

'When people ask me what brought you to psychedelics, I say, "Death." ... Death brought me to psychedelics.'

As far back as she can remember, Marg Ross had been interested in death.

When she was seven years old, her maternal grandmother died. She came from a family that didn't talk about things like death. Children were shut out of the grief process. All Ross knew was that her Nan was gone, buried in the ground, and that was that. But the questions had persisted: not only what happens when you die, but why don't people *talk* about death?

A few years later, her mum caught her with a bag of books from the library, all about death. Of course her mum had some questions, but the conversation turned to one of those stories a parent tells a child that permanently burrows into the child's mind, influencing their life for years to come.

Ross grew up in a small country town; one of those towns where the main street was really only the main street everyone inhabited. One day a horrific tragedy had engulfed the town. A house fire took the life of a three-year-old. Some time after the tragic event, Ross's mum saw the deceased child's mother on the main street. She crossed the road and rushed up to the mother.

'How are you going? Are you okay?' she asked.

The woman was so thankful for being approached. 'People are crossing the street to avoid talking to me. They don't know what to say.'

'So my mum would go and spend time with her,' Ross recalls. 'She'd cook her casseroles and be with her in grief. And Mum said, "Don't ever leave people when they need companionship – whether they're dying, whether they've just lost someone." And I never forgot that.

'It was formed very early in me, this wish to be witness or be present with people who were on the precipice of life and death, or had witnessed profound loss, because we edit it out of life. We edit death.'

All this led Ross into the field of clinical psychology – and after having a near-death experience herself in her late twenties, she ended up working with terminal cancer patients suffering from end-of-life anxiety at St Vincent's Hospital in Melbourne. Over several years, as she watched patients die filled with existential angst and terror, Ross started looking outside of the mainstream for ways of dealing with death. There had to be a better way, she thought.

Her research led her to the work of a US-based psychologist named Bill Richards (not the same William Richards who was a psychedelic psychiatrist in Melbourne in the 1960s). Back in the heyday of psychedelic medicine, Bill Richards had been among the first clinicians to explore the effect of psychedelics on terminally ill patients experiencing anxiety. After spending decades in limbo during the psychedelic research freeze across the 1970s, '80s and '90s, Richards started work again with Roland Griffiths in the 2000s as part of the big psychedelic renaissance at Johns Hopkins University in Baltimore.

In 2017, looking for more local answers, Ross saw that the EGA outdoor conference was coming up and decided to go. Over that weekend she went from knowing absolutely no one at the event to making some new friends that are still some of her closest. And there she found herself in the audience listening to Martin Williams give a talk about the dire state of psychedelic medicine in Australia.

As the conference progressed, Ross slowly felt a knot in her stomach grow tighter and tighter. She kept waiting to hear a presentation talking about someone getting a psychedelic trial off the ground in Australia but it never came. She thought, 'I think I can do this. Am I going to have to be the one that kicks it all off?' Back in her training days, Ross had had some experience with clinical trial coordination and she suspected she could get things over the line at her hospital.

A few weeks passed and Ross found herself at the start of 2018 sitting in front of her laptop facing a classic sliding doors moment. She was planning on leaving her job at St Vincent's Hospital, moving up north to work with a friend. 'Should I email my friend and get that plan going?' she wondered. Or should she send a quick email to that PRISM guy she'd met at EGA and see if he was keen on getting a trial in Australia going?

'Let's see what happens,' Ross thought, and she innocuously emailed Martin Williams. Within 24 hours, the two had met up for a coffee and started scribbling down notes on napkins. Australia's first psychedelic clinical trial had been born.

'DYING PATIENTS TO BE TREATED WITH MAGIC MUSHROOMS'

For about nine months, Ross and Williams worked on building up a robust clinical trial protocol. Not only was the trial set to be the first legal psychedelic research in Australia in decades, but Ross and Williams were looking to test something no one else in the world had yet explored.

The trial was to focus on using the drug psilocybin but, unlike previous end-of-life psychedelic trials in the United States focusing solely on patients with forms of advanced cancer, this study would look at a variety of participants with different terminal diseases. This included patients with advanced heart disease, motor neurone disease and severe kidney failure. The research team wanted to investigate psilocybin as a general palliative care tool.

Ross and Williams took their time building up a huge body of data. They talked to other researchers around the world and generated a collection of evidence that no hospital board or ethics body could deny. Ross also started to recruit a team of supporters inside the hospital. First, she needed a therapist partner.

All modern psychedelic medicine to date has been delivered by pairs of therapists. Having two therapists present during a drug session confers a variety of benefits. If someone needs to step out of the room for a moment, the patient won't be left alone, for example. Plus, having a pair of observers helps stave off any problems of inappropriate behaviour that could occur between an intoxicated patient and a potentially predatory therapist.

So Ross went to her head of department at St Vincent's, a psychiatrist named Justin Dwyer. She asked him, hesitantly: could they do this? Dwyer quietly studied the evidence and was convinced. He was on board. Next step was to get the sign-off from the hospital's head of palliative care. He also was impressed and supportive. Then the hospital's executive director, and another tick of support.

And finally, the big day came: delivering the application to the hospital's ethics board. This was the final nerve-racking moment, when all past attempts to get a psychedelic trial in Australia rolling had failed.

Suddenly, unexpectedly, the board gave the trial immediate conditional approval, seeing limited risk in testing the drugs in more terminally ill patients. It was September 2018, less than a year after the EGA conference that had started everything for Marg Ross.

From that moment, life for Ross and her team became all about the minutiae of running a clinical trial. But this wasn't a regular clinical trial. A whole truckload of extra work gets lobbed onto a study that involves highly scheduled drugs. And these were questions that had never been resolved within an Australian research context. Where do you even get pure psilocybin? Who makes it? How do you store it?

On top of that, when the hospital media unit got wind of the study being approved, a decision was made to get ahead of any negative stories in the press. This meant Ross would have to step in front of news cameras, months before the trial had even started. And once the story got out into the wild in early 2019, things started to get really chaotic.

It began with an article in one of Australia's most conservative newspapers. Ross thought it would just be a small article, maybe 20 pages deep into the day's paper. But no; it turned out to be a front-page 'exclusive': 'Dying patients will be treated with synthetic "magic mushrooms" in a Melbourne medical trial that aims to ease the paralysing anxiety felt by many who are in palliative care.'[30]

Suddenly Ross and the hospital were all over every Australian media outlet. The next day an impromptu news conference was held at the hospital. All the major TV news outlets were there. Ross was getting phone calls for interviews at all times of the day. Then things went international. The psychedelic community on Twitter blew the story up and Ross started receiving messages from all over the world. People from as far as Iceland and South Africa were wanting to talk.

'We were just these little nobodies, and nothing had changed,' Ross laughs, recalling those hectic weeks. 'We were just still this tiny little team. We're getting hammered with emails and people ringing, trying to get through and chat with us. Meanwhile, I'm just on the wards trying to do my day-to-day work.'

The wave of communication wasn't just from the media. Ross was also flooded with messages from desperate patients – people suffering from trauma, seeing no solution.

'It was horrible,' Ross tells me. 'In the beginning I would respond to every one of them, but it was just too much. I was becoming like a professional emailer. And it was awful. Harrowing stories. People were desperate.'

Then the emails began to turn demanding. People were threatening self-harm if they weren't let into the trial. Ross quickly went back to the hospital's ethics board looking for a way to manage it without having the whole trial fall apart. Reluctantly, she built walls around herself, putting an automated reply onto her email directing people to helplines, doctors, and other places that could manage their queries and concerns.

Time passed, the whirlwind settled, and the team got back to the real work of getting this trial started. Come early 2020, things were ready for launch. The first patient to be treated arrived at the dose site. Ross and Dwyer were ready to deliver their very first psilocybin treatment, and the first to be legally administered in Australia in nearly 50 years.

'Beautiful' and 'emotional' are the two words Ross uses to describe the landmark session. And that was that. Australia's first psychedelic clinical trial was underway.

Until ...

> We did another two sessions, and the final one was unbelievable and extraordinary. It was on a Friday in March; I'll never forget it. And Justin and I were just kind of blown away by what our participant was experiencing.
>
> Then the directives came in from the hospital. That afternoon. The patient went back and thankfully made it

home over the border. All of a sudden we were on the ward in scrubs and our trial had been suspended. About 85 per cent of non-Covid related research was ceased or halted.

The pandemic stopped everything in its tracks. All the momentum of the past few years; all the work, the planning, the legalities. The trial hit pause and didn't resume until nearly a year later, in February 2021.

'RELIGIOUS FERVOUR'

By the time Ross and Dwyer got their trial going again, it was clear the cultural landscape had dramatically changed. The tenor surrounding psychedelic medicine in Australia had shifted. Several other psychedelic clinical trials around the country were now in the works, and in March 2021 the Australian government surprised everyone by opening up a $15 million dollar funding round looking to 'kickstart' clinical trials using psychedelics for a variety of mental health disorders.[31] It was a boom time for psychedelic science in Australia.

Looking back, Ross notes how strange the overall cultural response was to her trial. When things were kicking off in 2019 and 2020, she was prepared to hit back against all the anti-drug prohibitionists. She had her arguments ready to counter any conservative calls of the research being unethical or dangerous. The talking points were primed.

But that pushback never came. Not once did Ross get to use the prepared defences of her research. Instead, she was stunned at how far the pendulum had swung in the other direction. 'It just went the other way. It was religious fervour,' Ross told me, still with a tone of disbelief.

Instead of defending the veracity of the research, she ended up tempering a wave of evangelism. Suddenly psychedelics were being hailed as a cure-all for everything. 'Whoa, hang on a second,' she thought. 'We need to do a bit more research to understand things first.'

In the end, Ross's trial was small but significant. Out of the 35 participants she and Dwyer treated with psilocybin, only four were officially classified as 'non-responders'. These were patients who wholly hated the experience. In Ross's more informal words, 'They were just like, "Nope, not doing that again. That was fucking terrible!"'

But Ross's biggest takeaway from the trial has been how frustratingly complex and fraught the whole idea of studying psychedelics is. Her close contact with the patients in the trial revealed how our simplistic depression and anxiety scales often fundamentally miss what these unusual drugs are actually doing. For example, on paper, one of the non-responders in the trial looks like the study's biggest failure: a woman who, for around 48 hours after the psilocybin dose, felt like she wanted to die. Even though she entered the study with pre-existing feelings of suicide, the researchers had an ethical responsibility to report the days following the dose as an 'adverse event'.

However, months later, that patient's story looked very different. Ross says this woman ultimately was consumed with a sense of extraordinary calm. She started writing poetry, went back on antidepressants, and looked back on her psychedelic experience as profoundly transformative. Nevertheless, in the published study this participant is logged as non-responsive, suffering severe adverse effects from the treatment and nothing more. 'Psychedelics are not about symptom reduction,' Ross told me.

> [The drug] might do that by virtue of the fact that it's kind of bringing some personal transformation forward, but it's about transformation. And we are terrible at capturing that. We're using these really awful checklists: 'How did you feel today?' 'Well, actually, I saw my dead husband. I danced with him.' 'Oh, okay, but how did you sleep on a scale of one to ten?'
>
> Our study had great results. Yes, we reduced anxiety. Yes, we reduced depression. But we can do that with pills. You can dampen symptoms with a decent whack of sedative, but that's not getting to the core of it. What was transformational was that fear of death reduced; demoralisation reduced. Hopelessness was so low at the end it could almost not be detected statistically. Spiritual wellbeing went up, quality of life went up, and perspective shifted. How they faced mortality was extraordinary. So there's a big transformation going on.[32]

THE LETTERS

As the public face of Australia's first psychedelic clinical trial, Ross has received lots of strange bits of correspondence over the years. Of course there were the constant messages from people looking for tips on how to take 'magic mushrooms' for their health, and there were also weird little objects mailed in to the hospital. Many a massive self-published tome was sent to Ross, spruiking a person's individual journey through psychedelics.

But one day an unusual letter stopped Ross in her tracks.

It was a handwritten piece, in old-school, cursive copperplate. 'Dear Dr Ross,' it declared on the envelope; the handwriting was beautiful but a little shaky. This was clearly something meaningful penned by someone very old. Ross opened the letter and was speechless. It was from John Mackay, the notorious psychiatrist responsible for treating hundreds of psychedelic patients at Newhaven hospital in the 1960s.

'It was staggering. I'm like, "Oh my god. I've been contacted by a cult psychiatrist."'

Mackay congratulated Ross on her work, and offered support, encouragement and even some advice garnered from his expansive experience administering psychedelic drugs to patients. It was lovely, caring, sincere and deeply unsettling. In the back of Ross's mind, she said to herself, 'Don't get sucked in by this. Remember the brutality of what happened and the way this man harmed innumerable patients back in the day.'

Ross never directly responded to Mackay's letter but she did keep it. It sits in a frame in her home office, a reminder of how wild and strange it was to get this trial going and be thrust into the spotlight.

A second piece of correspondence Ross received was just as memorable, but for slightly different reasons. This time, it came in an email. Despite the onslaught of communications, she often delved into her messy inbox to read the thoughts and experiences people were sharing. This piece of correspondence began like many others: a person sharing a story of how certain psychedelic experiences in their youth changed their life. But something quickly caught Ross's eye. This woman said her first doses of psychedelics were given by psychiatrists at Newhaven.

'I'd heard many stories about the horrors of Newhaven. So I naturally braced myself for a harrowing story, but she didn't have the harrowing story I thought she was going to have.'

Instead, this woman spoke of a stunning multi-year journey with psychedelics and group therapy, beginning in 1964 and continuing until the early 1970s. The story moved from Newhaven to another hospital after cult activity emerged, and told a story of psychedelic healing over dozens of psilocybin sessions. It was wildly different to how psychedelic medicine was being practised in the 21st century.

The correspondent was in her early nineties, and the experiences she recounted were vivid, life-changing and incredibly lucid. Ross was surprised at how clearly these psychedelic encounters from more than 50 years ago were remembered and described. It was a glorious moment connecting the past, present and future of psychedelic medicine, an interaction that united Australia's earliest psychedelic medicine experiments with its newest iteration, separated by more than half a century of public silence and taboo.

That woman's name was Evelyn Harrison.

2

MAGIC MUSHROOMS

WHERE DOES PSILOCYBIN COME FROM, AND IS THAT ALL THERE IS?

'Some species of toadstool give rise to a kind of intoxication. A former colleague of mine told me how his parents ate once a dish of mushrooms, and as the meal progressed they gradually became more and more hilarious, the most simple remark giving rise to peals of laughter. The intoxication passed off without any unpleasant effects. Probably some poisonous kind had been included, possibly one of the dung-inhabiting species.'

John Burton Cleland, *Toadstools and Mushrooms and Other Larger Fungi of South Australia*, Government Printer, Adelaide, 1934, p. 19[1]

The group was tight. Only a couple of participants were first-timers, and Dee, who was leading the ceremony, had done this many times before. The night started like any other ceremony: some breathwork, sound healing. But by the end of the evening, one participant would be dead and another under suspicion of manslaughter.[2]

Rachael Dixon had been attending magic-mushroom sessions for around 18 months, and from all accounts was the happiest she'd been in years.[3] Her only son was grown up, successfully studying at university, and she was rekindling a decades-long dormant relationship with her ex-husband. For Rachael, the magic-mushroom sessions had been extraordinarily positive for her mental health and in April 2024 she was embarking on her sixth ceremony.

'She was fit, healthy and so happy,' her older sister recounted to a journalist. 'Rachael described this [sixth] therapy session as a homecoming and said it was the last time she was going to do it because she was going to get all the answers she wanted.'[4]

Rachael had known Deanne Matthews for almost eight years, having first connected with Dee to practise reiki. For a couple of years, Dee had been running what she called 'healing sessions', in which a group would convene and consume magic mushrooms with a focused therapeutic intent. The make-up of each group was different slightly from session to session. In the case of this session in April 2024, two of the nine participants were new. Days before a session the group always connected over Zoom to meet and discuss their intentions for the ceremony.

Kay* was one of the 'newbies' to the group that evening. It wasn't her first time taking part in a psychedelic medicine ceremony. She well knew how these things should play out, and to her everything seemed responsible and serious.

---

* This is a pseudonym, as the participant wishes to remain anonymous.

That particular evening Dee made only one announcement that was out of the ordinary. 'Tonight we're going to have subs,' she declared to everyone early on. Kay, who'd taken mushrooms recreationally before, immediately understood what Dee was referring to. *Psilocybe subaeruginosa,* informally referred to in psychedelic circles as 'subs', is a species of magic mushroom native to Australia and New Zealand. It's a fungus particularly prominent in the southern states of Australia, and it forms its unique mycelium network around wood debris. 'Subs' sit in contrast to a more commonly consumed species of magic mushroom, *Psilocybe cubensis.* Known as 'cubes', these mushrooms emerge from cow dung and in Australia are found mostly in the northern states.

After some preparatory rituals – smudging, cleanses, etc. – Dee moved around the circle with a bowl of magic mushrooms that had been ground into powder. Every participant was given the choice of how strong a dose they wanted to start with: 1, 2 or 3 grams. Dee precisely measured out each person's preferred dose using scales.

Time passed, everyone descended into their own trip, and Dee eventually went around the circle a second time to offer everyone another dose. Again, each participant was given a choice to take up to 3 grams more. Being an experienced tripper, Kay was all in, taking 6 grams all up across the two doses. This was a big dose, but Kay didn't do things by halves and she felt the environment was safe.

At this point the clearest timeline of events we have is from the coroner's report.[5] That document notes the first dose was given at 6.15 pm, and the second around 90 minutes later. Sometime around 11.30 pm Rachael called out for help. Dee went to Rachael and tried to move her outside for some fresh air, but as she stood up her legs just gave out.

Despite nearing the end of the trip, Kay and the rest of the circle were still miles away. Kay recounts being able to hear a bit of a ruckus but it was very distant. By midnight Dee was on the phone to emergency services. Rachael had stopped breathing. A first responder soon appeared with a defibrillator and at 12.09 am the first wave of paramedics arrived. Rachael's heart had stopped. The paramedics tried to resuscitate her for half an hour but to no avail. Rachael had passed away.

By that stage most participants had emerged from their trip. Everyone was sitting around the circle, unsure what was happening. More paramedics arrived, and then, according to Kay's recollections, everyone started 'dropping like flies'.

It began with one of the other 'newbies', a woman in her sixties.

'I can't feel my legs!' she cried out. A paramedic rushed over and started to collect her vital signs, and then the woman in the circle next to her was struck. 'I can't feel my legs either!' she said, alarmingly.

Kay was feeling fine at that point but couldn't really process what was unfolding. 'What the fuck is happening?' she thought.

A wave of panic spread among the paramedics. Was this mushroom poisoning? Did everyone need to get to hospital immediately? No one knew what was happening.

The two participants with leg paralysis were taken aside and the remaining members of the group tried to keep calm. Some food went around – soup and bread. Kay devoured it; food tastes extra good after a big mushroom journey. Then she started eating a muffin. As she chewed the muffin, her jaw suddenly locked up. A wave of numbness quickly spread across her entire face. She couldn't swallow, move her tongue, anything. Her face was frozen.

Almost choking, Kay cried out to a paramedic with a muffled, 'Help me.' The medic rushed over and noted with familiarity that Kay wasn't the first of the group to show this symptom. Five minutes passed, and Kay tried to calm herself. Feeling slowly returned to her face. The paramedic moved on.

Kay started eating, and again her face just flopped with a weird kind of sudden muscle weakness. What was happening? She stayed calm, breathed through it, and feeling quickly returned.

The paramedics ended up taking the first two paralysis victims to hospital. The rest of the group stayed. Over the next few hours, everyone felt some kind of paralytic body wave after the mushrooms. For some it was an odd weakness in their legs when trying to walk. Others had trouble swallowing for short periods of time.

The next day everyone was shaken. Rachael had died. The police were involved. An investigation was inevitable. But what had happened?

Dee was an experienced and well-regarded facilitator. Despite early hyperbolic media reports, this wasn't a case of someone simply picking the wrong type of mushrooms. After all, if this were a conventional case of mushroom poisoning it wouldn't have happened so quickly, and everyone else in the circle would have been in massive trouble. The mushrooms everyone consumed were definitely psychedelic. Everyone had a trip.

On the Sunday morning Kay called the friend who was meant to accompany her on the trip but had pulled out at the last moment. Upon hearing the story, the friend, who had some knowledge of magic mushrooms and psychedelic science, immediately responded with, 'I reckon that sounds like wood-lover paralysis.'

'What?' Kay asked.

After finishing the call, Kay turned to Dee. 'A friend of mine suggested what could have happened was something called wood-lover paralysis,' Kay told her. Dee said she had heard murmurings of the phenomenon but couldn't be sure that was what happened.

When Kay got home she started researching and dropped down a massive rabbit hole. What was wood-lover paralysis? What was in certain magic mushrooms that could be causing this? Could the phenomenon be responsible for Rachael's death? And was this ceremony the first time wood-lover paralysis had been seen and recorded in a group context?

HOFMANN GOT IT WRONG

Modern science has focused on psilocybin as the primary psychoactive compound in magic mushrooms for more than 50 years. However, the phenomenon of wood-lover paralysis suggests there could be other molecules in some magic mushrooms we have been missing. As we'll soon learn, scientists have recently discovered an unexpected variety of potentially psychoactive compounds in magic mushrooms. Wood-lover paralysis is perhaps the most powerful clue we have that there could be other molecules yet to be catalogued, and the more researchers uncover, the more complex our understanding of psychedelics gets. But how did we miss this complexity for so long?

The persistent, almost monomaniacal focus on psilocybin is intertwined with the one story that has dominated the narrative of magic mushrooms in recent Western culture. If you have read any popular account of magic mushrooms you are likely to know the tale of R Gordon Wasson, the investment banker who, in the 1950s, became obsessed with finding the mysterious 'God's flesh' mushroom.

Since the 16th century, tales had swirled of this special mushroom used in ancient religious ceremony, but no Westerner had been able to find it. After several trips to Mexico, Wasson finally found what he was looking for. When he published an iconic article in *Life* magazine in 1957 titled 'Seeking the Magic Mushroom', the novel psychedelic crashed into the mainstream.

Perhaps a lesser-known note to the tale is that of the CIA's hunt for this mysterious mushroom across the same time period.

At the height of Cold War paranoia, the US spy agency was looking for any way to get ahead of the Soviets, and developing unique mind-controlling drugs was one strategy. An organic chemist named John Moore was recruited by the CIA to hunt down this special mushroom.[6] In mid-1955 Moore got word that Wasson had potentially found the Holy Grail. He got in touch with Wasson and helped fund the next expedition to Mexico to get samples of these mushrooms.

So, Wasson's iconic expedition to gather the first ever confirmed samples of magic mushrooms was surreptitiously funded by the CIA. And not only that, upon returning to the United States, Moore took his share of the samples to work on identifying the key psychoactive components. The CIA wanted their new mind-control drug. But homing in on what chemicals in the mushroom were causing the hallucinogenic effects turned out to be harder than anyone had imagined.

A French botanist named Roger Heim was working with Wasson at the time on the same investigation; however, his team in Paris couldn't crack the mystery. Samples of the mushrooms were then sent to a couple of big pharmaceutical companies in the US. Chemists at Merck and at Smith, Kline & French couldn't figure it out. Then finally Heim and Wasson looked to the labs at pharmaceutical company Sandoz in Switzerland. After all, these guys were working with LSD and had some familiarity with psychedelic chemicals.

Albert Hofmann, the 'father of LSD', jumped at the chance to solve this strange chemistry mystery, but much like the researchers at other labs, he quickly hit a brick wall. All the cursory animal tests designed to detect potential psychoactive extracts from the mushrooms led to nothing. Hofmann wondered whether the psychedelic element at work was similar to LSD, insofar as its hallucinogenic effects weren't immediately apparent in non-human studies. So, Hofmann did what he'd done over a decade earlier with LSD: he tested the mushrooms on himself.

For about six hours, Hofmann experienced a deeply vivid swirl of psychedelic imagery, all tinged with Mexican characteristics. He associated the distinctive cultural thematics of the trip to the fact he knew the mushrooms were from Mexico and were used there ceremonially. From here, Hofmann and his team knew the mushrooms were psychoactive and they then proceeded to isolate, concentrate and name two specific chemicals: psilocybin and psilocin.

Summing up his achievement several decades later in his autobiography, Hofmann wrote:

> Thus with the isolation and synthesis of the active principles, the demystification of the magic mushrooms was accomplished. The compounds whose wondrous effects led the Indians to believe for millennia that a god was residing in the mushrooms had their chemical structures elucidated and could be produced synthetically in flasks.[7]

Sandoz swiftly commercialised psilocybin, branding it Indocybin and selling it to psychiatrists around the world. It was marketed as an effective adjunct to psychotherapy, much like LSD but shorter acting. John Moore had been beaten to the punch but that didn't dissuade him or the CIA from their plans. They simply just became loyal Sandoz customers, buying psilocybin and starting their experiments to turn it into a spy weapon. Unsurprisingly, the CIA experiments failed; they discovered that psilocybin, much like LSD, was not at all helpful in mind-control pursuits.

In hindsight, Hofmann's initial chemistry work with magic mushrooms was mostly accurate. He was correct in identifying psilocybin as the main psychoactive chemical in magic mushrooms. But he also got some things wrong.

For example, his initial speculations around the way mushrooms biosynthesised psilocybin were way off the mark.[8] And this small technical mistake led to decades of misunderstanding around what chemicals were actually in magic mushrooms.

For years scientists knew magic mushrooms produced psilocybin by starting with a molecule called tryptophan, a key amino acid. But exactly how the fungi did this was unknown. Hofmann's initial biosynthesis hypothesis was wrong. He overlooked a number of active chemicals in magic mushrooms and it wasn't until well into the 21st century that researchers finally understood how psilocybin was produced. And in that understanding emerged a whole new idea.

What if some of these other molecules could influence the psychoactive properties of magic mushrooms? Had we been missing something all these years? Could the 'trip' from magic mushrooms be more than just psilocybin?

'I CANNOT FUCKING WALK'

As a medical doctor with a strong interest in harm minimisation, Simon Beck's curiosity was piqued in the late 2010s when he heard the story of a friend who experienced a terrifying bout of paralysis after taking a handful of magic mushrooms. This friend was an experienced Australian psychonaut who knew how to correctly identify local magic mushrooms. This wasn't merely a case of someone picking the wrong type of mushroom. And the patch the mushrooms came from was in a completely natural, forested location, so there was no chance the fungi had been inadvertently sprayed with some kind of pesticide or toxin.

Beck's research instinct kicked in, and he started digging through decades of mycology literature to see if this phenomenon had ever been reported. Barely a handful of references to anything like what his friend had experienced could be found. The earliest mention of something even close was in a Japanese mycology journal. Published in 1973, the report detailed several 'hallucinogenic mushroom poisonings', citing three instances of users experiencing 'intermittent paralysis of the limbs'.[9]

Fast forward nearly 20 years to the 1990s, when an article published in the *Journal of Psychoactive Drugs* comprehensively reviewed psychedelic mushrooms in Australia and New Zealand, and chronicled a substantial number of case reports of mushroom poisoning.[10] Almost all the reports in the article consisted of cases where a mushroom user presented with discomforting psychological effects after consuming the drug. But one small section near the end discussed strange physical effects.

One of the article's co-authors, New Zealand psychiatrist Karl Jansen, attended the home of a person in distress after consuming magic mushrooms. The subject was experiencing profound muscle weakness and shortness of breath. The person was monitored closely, with signs of muscle weakness persisting for more than 18 hours after all psychedelic effects had dissipated. Jansen reported several other cases of similar paralysis, which all seemed to occur in people who had picked magic mushrooms from the same spot:

> Others ingesting the mushrooms from this paddock also suffered various forms of muscle weakness (e.g., lazy eyelid, which is extremely unlikely to have a psychological origin), extending in all cases for many hours beyond the end of the change in consciousness. In several cases, strong and robust men who had extensive experience with psychedelic drugs collapsed while crossing the road due

to severe muscle weakness – a potentially life-threatening situation.[11]

In the article, Jansen and his co-authors present this story as unequivocally the result of mushrooms being sprayed with some kind of agricultural fungicide. However, this is offered without any evidence beyond a mere presumption that the spraying of wild mushrooms had been occurring in the country. After all, what else could explain such an odd, toxic, phenomenon?

A few years later, influential US mycologist Paul Stamets made a brief mention of mushroom-induced paralysis in his iconic book *Psilocybin Mushrooms of the World*.[12] When discussing several wood-loving species of psilocybin mushroom, Stamets suggests there are some reports of people losing muscle control. But this phenomenon is quickly hand-waved away as a rare mystery for another time.

Other than these few scattered references to an unexplained type of muscle weakness, Simon Beck couldn't find any serious investigation of the phenomenon in scientific literature. More online research led him to one of the infamous parts of the internet: an online forum called Shroomery.

Back in the 1990s, psychedelic culture thrived on the internet. The emergence of such a novel technology propagated an incredible array of new information-sharing. Websites like Erowid and Lycaeum connected psychedelic communities around the globe. Knowledge that previously was guarded or hard to discover suddenly became available to anyone with a modem. The internet's influence on psychedelic culture was akin to throwing fuel on a tiny fire. A culture that had been quietly percolating in disconnected bubbles for decades blew up with a wild force.

In 1997, Ythan Bernstein was on his school summer break and looking for information on psychedelic mushrooms. The 15-year-old was adept at surfing the early internet and soon noticed how hard it was to get good, reliable information on mushrooms. So he started up his own website called Shroomery. The site quickly became a hub for knowledge-sharing, with psychedelic mycologists around the world passing on experiences and expertise. It also slowly revealed many mushroom users reporting strange bouts of muscle weakness following the consumption of certain species of magic mushrooms.[13]

As mentioned in passing by Stamets all those years before, the phenomenon only seemed to occur with a few particular wood-loving species of psilocybin mushroom – and even then it seemed to be rare, and isolated to specific patches. The earliest reference Beck could find to the phenomenon on Shroomery forums was a post from 2001 titled 'I cannot fucking walk'.

The author recounted an experience being unable to walk after taking a moderate dose of a mushroom species known as *Psilocybe azurescens*. The species is mostly found in woody environments along the west coast of the United States. Recent genetic studies hypothesise *P. azurescens* to be closely related to Australia's *P. subaeruginosa* ('subs'), or even possibly the same species.

The few brief responses to the post on Shroomery at the time speculated about what could have caused the muscle weakness. Maybe it was something to do with the preparation method? Maybe it was a random unidentified molecule? Either way, most members on the forum agreed this was an exceptionally rare phenomenon.

A handful more cases on the topic were posted over the next few years, and a 2009 post called 'Mushroom Paralysis (Wood Lovers)' essentially coined the name that subsequently stuck with the condition.[14] From then it was generally referred to as 'wood-lover paralysis': an unusually rare and strange thing that occasionally happens with some species of magic mushrooms that grow in woody environments.

SIMON BECK'S CURIOSITY WAS NOT SATIATED. MOST of these forum reports were from the United States, but surely this was happening here in Australia too? After all, 'subs' are ubiquitous wood-loving magic mushrooms found all over the east and south of the country.

This was early 2020, and magic-mushroom use was not nearly as rare as it had been in the past. Psychedelic renaissance stories were all over the media. Even Netflix had its share of documentaries touting the miracles of mushrooms. So Beck decided to put a call out for paralysis experiences on a Facebook forum with a relatively large community of psilocybin mushroom enthusiasts from Australia and New Zealand. He framed the post as a public safety announcement, describing the phenomenon in a 'be alert, not alarmed' way.

The response was unexpected. Scores of community members started sharing similar experiences, thanking Beck for airing something many had never talked about.

'Yep happened to me and a couple of mates, first time ever, very bizarre experience.'

'A friend of mine had their jaw and legs stop working, they kept falling over and couldn't talk or stand for the duration of the day.'

'Yep been there. Couldn't eat my nachos. Jaw felt like it was disjointed. Couldn't walk. Couldn't unlock my car with the key cos hands were like claws and just wouldn't work.'

'Oh, shit. This explains a trip I had years ago, experienced something very similar. Scared me off shrooms for a couple of years.'

'Have had it for the first time a few weeks ago; it was unexpected (because I never had it before, so thought I was "immune" to it) and intermittent – it came and went away several times.'

'Experienced this last week from Subs picked wild then dried. My friend and I were both affected pretty badly. Considering we were 8 floors up in an abandoned building we were screwed and had to wait for a friend to come and rescue us. Started out as just a strange numb feeling in face and progressed to legs, arms, and my friend said his neck and breathing were affected too. Got kinda scary. Antihistamines didn't work, but the effect wore off over the next 12 hours or so.'

Joining forces with the Australian mycology expert Caine Barlow, Beck drafted a survey in the hopes of trying to understand how prevalent this mysterious condition actually was. 'I was quite worried about the potential risks,' Beck explained to me. 'I could see the potential for accidents and could certainly see the potential for some respiratory depression as well. We decided the best way to get some basic information would be to actually get a clearer understanding of how it presents.' From there, Beck and Barlow could look into the individual and environmental factors that might play a role.

The way the condition seemed to come out of nowhere concerned Beck. What if someone took magic mushrooms, decided to go for a swim, and, while out in the ocean, was suddenly overcome with muscle weakness? If they drowned, how would we even know what the cause was?

The survey was open for a relatively short time but the volume of responses shocked Beck and Barlow. Around 400 people responded, with roughly 165 reporting clear instances of wood-lover paralysis. Pretty quickly, the pair of citizen science researchers got a clear and unprecedented picture of the condition, and several common theories immediately went out the window.

Wood-lover paralysis was not related to environmental toxins. Survey participants reported picking their mushrooms from a broad assortment of locations, from isolated, unmanaged national parks and state forests, to lands adjacent to farms. There was no way a single agricultural chemical could have infiltrated such a diverse array of places. This wasn't caused by a foreign chemical or pesticide.

What about individual allergies or medication interactions? Nope, that didn't fit either. The sheer variety of responses knocked that hypothesis out the window too.

Beck is, however, open to the limitations of his original 2020 survey. He understands how informal and narrow it was. 'The feedback we got from our first submission to a journal is that, "Well, how do you know it's not psychosomatic? How do you know this isn't just the psychedelic effect?"' Here Beck and Barlow faced perhaps the most challenging stigma often thrown at psychonauts. Beck suggests that anyone familiar with psychedelics will understand how preposterous the question is, but countering it with more objective data is a little trickier. Were people just tripping so hard they felt like their body was paralysed?

Pharmacologically, Beck argues the fact that the residual weakness from wood-lover paralysis seems to last for days is a good sign this is something other than just the psychological effects of psilocybin. Also, and probably most telling, is the fact that this phenomenon only happens with certain wood-loving species of psilocybin mushrooms.

'Cubes don't do it,' Beck adds. No one is reporting experiences of muscle weakness or paralysis with other species of magic mushrooms.

Okay. The duo was comfortable declaring wood-lover paralysis a real phenomenon. The survey established something was certainly going on.

Now what?

THE END OF THE DINOSAURS, THE BEGINNING OF PSILOCYBIN

To understand exactly what could be causing wood-lover paralysis, we need to pause for a moment and understand how psilocybin exists in nature in the first place. And to do that we need to go back in time – to the age of the dinosaurs.

Fungi, and mushrooms, have been around for hundreds of millions of years but psilocybin only appeared around 66 million years ago.[15] Canny readers will likely notice the relevance of that date. This was around the time of what has been called the K–Pg extinction event: the infamous transition from the Cretaceous period to the Paleogene, precipitated by a massive catastrophic disaster that resulted in not only the end of the dinosaurs, but the extinction of more than 90 per cent of all mammal species on the planet.[16]

But how did the death of the dinosaurs coincide with the evolution of psilocybin?

The strongest theory we have is a huge asteroid smashed into our planet, landing in what we now know as the Yucatán Peninsula, around south-east Mexico. The asteroid was at least 10 kilometres wide and left a crater with a diameter of 200 kilometres. The impact devastated almost all life on Earth. Any living thing near the impact was immediately vaporised, but the secondary effects of the calamity rippled across the globe. Giant tsunamis, raging wildfires, mega-earthquakes. Vaporised rock in the air caused sulphuric acid rain, killing off vast volumes of marine life.

Anything surviving the acute effects of the impact was left facing a transformed and dying world. Billions of tonnes of soot and silt settled in the upper atmosphere, blocking all sunlight. Recent estimates suggest it took at least 18 months for enough light to return to the surface to allow plants to photosynthesise.[17] Plants, trees and animals all perished.

But this wasn't an apocalypse for every organism on the planet.

In particular, two types of life thrived in this post-impact catastrophe: fungi and gastropods.[18] The enormous volume of decomposing organic matter was like an orgiastic all-you-can-eat buffet for slugs, snails and fungi.

We know gastropods were flourishing at this point in history. And we know wood-decomposing fungi would have been deeply nourished by all the dying plant matter. It was under these conditions that fungi developed the ability to biosynthesise psilocybin. But why then? What function could this molecule serve fungi?

Everything gets extra-speculative from here, but I had a head-spinning conversation with mycologist Caine Barlow, who helped me understand the history of magic mushrooms, and he succinctly summed up the competing hypotheses underpinning the emergence of psilocybin.

'There's two viewpoints on this: to either stop predation of the mushroom or, perhaps in some cases, to attract predation of the mushroom,' Caine explained. 'So a predator eats the mushroom and then spreads the spores, or psilocybin actively stops predation of the mushroom while it grows.'

Psilocybin isn't explicitly toxic to most gastropods. So its role couldn't have been a poison in the traditional sense, but rather the molecule possibly served to manipulate the behaviour of a predator to help disperse its spores. Because the shape of psilocybin molecules resemble that of the common neurotransmitter serotonin, it can influence a broad range of physiological processes. In gastropods, for example, serotonin is known to play a role in locomotion, appetite and reproduction.

One mycologist I spoke to recounted a story where a colleague informally experimented with feeding slugs magic mushrooms. The slugs suddenly switched from nocturnal behaviours to being much more active during the day. This researcher speculated psilocybin was potentially influencing the way gastropods sense light, triggering more constant activity and movement across the day. Why would this be useful to the fungi? Well, disorientating the slug could make it more susceptible to predation. And fungi spores are remarkably resilient when travelling through the guts of both gastropods and the animals that eat gastropods.

Maybe psilocybin was evolutionarily advantageous to some mushrooms? The slug eats the mushroom. The psilocybin makes the slug more active during daylight hours. That activity makes it easier for predators to catch the slug. This heightened predation thus spreads the mushroom's spores further.

In a post-apocalyptic world filled with flourishing volumes of fungi and gastropods, it was likely very useful for some species of mushroom to develop novel and advantageous ways of spreading their spores. For whatever reason, psilocybin turned out to be a profoundly useful mutation that not only persisted in various species of fungi but ultimately thrived.

This initial emergence of psilocybin in fungi was in a highly specific environmental niche. However, as time passed, the molecule proved just as useful to fungi in other conditions. And here scientists have tracked several divergences in the family tree of psilocybin-producing fungi. Over millions of years fungi picked up new tricks, shifting from using decomposing wood as their home, to soil, and then to animal dung. But as well as ancestral sharing of psilocybin-producing genes, scientists found a few mushroom species picked up the ability to produce psilocybin through a curious process called horizontal gene transfer.

As the name suggests, horizontal gene transfer occurs when genes are shared between two different species that likely lived in relatively close confines. Exactly how this process takes place in fungi is a bit mysterious but the best guess is bacteria in the environment pick up certain genes and transfer them to other species of fungi. This is a long, slow process, but the fact that geneticists have been able to track these gene transfer events in fungi suggests psilocybin is a very useful molecule for mushrooms in certain environmental niches.

CUBES ARE CUBES

All of this ultimately brings us to perhaps the most well-known species of magic mushroom, *Psilocybe cubensis*. When most people talk about magic mushrooms, it's a good bet they are referring to *P. cubensis*, also known as 'cubes'. This species of psilocybin-producing mushroom emerged anywhere from 10 to 25 million years ago and is famous for growing in animal dung. Unlike older species of fungi that develop long-standing mycelial networks underground in soil or in decomposing wood, cubes live more symbiotically with mammals. The mushrooms are eaten by animals, spores are excreted, and then a new generation of mushrooms grows from the dung. This cycle of life has perhaps been amplified by the human domestication of livestock. So humans probably came into frequent contact with cubes as the fungi drifted towards inhabiting the dung of cows and other similar domesticated animals.

In the end, this is one of the reasons why cubes are the best-known magic mushroom to humans. Alongside this, *P. cubensis* is easy to grow for the home mycologist and was solidly entrenched into Western psychedelic culture by the publication of a book titled *Psilocybin: Magic Mushroom Grower's Guide* in the 1970s.[19] This now-iconic book was authored by the McKenna brothers (Terence and Dennis), a pair of psychonauts and ethnobotanists whose profound experiences with magic mushrooms in the Amazon rainforest led them to drive a wave of psychedelic culture in the 1980s and '90s.

A common saying in the psychedelic community is 'cubes are cubes'. This refers to the tendency of *P. cubensis* mushrooms to deliver relatively consistent trip experiences. While certain mycologists have cultivated novel strains of the species, it's thought these only really differ in terms of psilocybin potency. Some unique cultivated strains of cubes do contain exceptionally high concentrations of psilocybin, so the variety of subjective effects between different magic mushrooms is thought to come down to three factors: dose, set (the mindset of a user going into an experience) and setting (the environmental setting of an experience).

Cubes are cubes.

Over the years, however, researchers have gradually discovered there may be more to magic mushrooms than just psilocybin. In fact it wasn't until 2017 that we fully understood exactly how mushrooms actually make psilocybin. And alongside this landmark discovery came the realisation that there is a lot more going on inside these fungi than we thought.

THE PSILOCYBIN GENE CLUSTER

Psilocybin starts with one crucial building block used by all forms of life – an amino acid called tryptophan. Our own bodies use tryptophan, ingested through dietary sources, to generate a whole assortment of critical neurotransmitters and hormones. Psilocybin-producing mushrooms have an extraordinary ability to synthesise tryptophan internally, using the amino acid as a scaffold for a number of different uses.

Back in the 1950s Albert Hofmann was correct when

he hypothesised tryptophan to be the first step in the magic mushroom's process to create psilocybin. That first step involves a tweak to the tryptophan molecule, turning it into a different kind of molecule we call a tryptamine. From here Hofmann could only speculate through the potential steps that ended up with the psilocybin molecule. He presumed the process involved transforming the tryptamine molecule into something similar to what we know of as the neurotransmitter serotonin. And from there, just a couple of molecular tweaks took you to psilocybin.[20]

It was a predictable procedure, stepping through a series of intermediate molecules that were relatively well-known to scientists. A little over 50 years later we realised Hofmann had missed a few things.

From a trio of pharmacologists in Germany, a niche 2017 paper titled 'Enzymatic Synthesis of Psilocybin' changed the world of psychedelic mushrooms for a small community of scientists.[21] The research finally solved the mystery of psilocybin biosynthesis, identifying four key genes that produce the psychoactive chemical: PsiD, PsiK, PsiM and PsiH. Subsequently known as the psilocybin gene cluster, these four genes produce specific enzymes that the mushrooms use to convert the amino acid tryptophan into psilocybin.

The research revealed this to be a very efficient step-by-step process, with each enzyme tweaking the previous molecule to ultimately end up with psilocybin. Some of the molecules created along the way, like baeocystin, had previously been discovered in a few species of magic mushroom, but this new research demonstrated exactly how a cluster of four genes produce this variety of tryptamines.

Perhaps most significantly, the discovery suggested it was possible for different magic mushrooms to contain various combinations of these other tryptamine metabolites, depending on the characteristics of the gene cluster.

But a big hole in the research at this point was the fact that, so far, there had been almost no work looking into the potential genetic diversity of wild magic mushrooms. Could this psilocybin gene cluster present differently in different species of magic mushrooms?

PICTURE STEVE IRWIN, BUT INSTEAD OF WRESTLING crocodiles he developed an interest in mushroom genetics. This is the most succinct way I can describe Queenslander Alistair McTaggart, whose bracingly engaging mix of Aussie friendliness and hard genetic science can sometimes feel surreal in conversation. ('Whoa mate, check out the allelic diversity in that psilocybin gene cluster ... that's unreal!')

McTaggart's story, like many in this book, was dramatically shaped by Covid. When the pandemic hit in 2020, he faced an existential crisis. Like many plants he studied in evolutionary biology, he had specialised himself into such a specific niche he wasn't sure there was a place for him in any broad academic ecosystem. Mycology, molecular biology, fungal reproduction, population genomics – all highly particular, disparate corners of science.

What was he to do? Why not try to fill a gap in the scientific record? He had access to a lab and resources through his job at the University of Queensland, so why not try to record the genomes of as many Australian magic mushrooms as he could gather?

Maybe it was naivety that got him over the line. He didn't really know what he was getting himself into. Even the very first step of the process was a mystery to him: who do you contact to get permission to work with magic mushrooms? Eventually McTaggart focused on the Queensland Department of Health as the body that regulates whether someone can get a permit to work with illegal materials such as magic mushrooms. There was an application; 'Let's fill it out and see what happens,' he thought. In what was a surprise to absolutely everyone, his application was approved and McTaggart unexpectedly became the first person to get a permit to legally work with, and grow, magic mushrooms in a lab in Australia.

Time was of the essence. His contract at UQ was limited so he needed to move fast. Now he needed samples, and lots of them. Luckily the Australian mycology underground caught wind of his work and the grapevine sparked up. Connections were made and more than a dozen citizen scientists around the country started gathering mushroom spore samples to send to Queensland for analysis.

It was a stunningly unique project, initially running on the smell of an oily rag. There was no funding in that first year, and genetic sequencing isn't a cheap process. Just screening the genome of one sample could cost hundreds of dollars. And to do a good population study McTaggart would need at least 100 genomes.

In a moment of synchronicity, a burst of funding shot through the project to give it a lifeline. Called the Australian Functional Fungi Initiative, the money came from a non-profit research group called Bioplatforms Australia. That group was funded by the Australian government. Thanks, government funding!

Alongside the academic value of gathering such a unique genomic dataset, McTaggart had a couple of big-picture questions he wanted to answer. The first was: when did *Psilocybe cubensis* actually get to Australia?

His genetic findings for *P. cubensis* were interesting, albeit unsurprising. McTaggart's research revealed, for the first time, these dung-inhabiting mushrooms were introduced into Australia around a century ago – give or take a few decades.[22] The mushrooms likely arrived via cattle transports but exactly where they came from is still unknown. South Africa or India are McTaggart's two best guesses at this point.

In terms of genetic diversity around the psilocybin gene cluster, the research also found most cubes were remarkably similar. All cubes presented with just one copy of each psilocybin-producing gene. Cultivated varieties, such as those strains grown domestically since the McKenna manual in the 1970s, displayed low levels of genetic diversity. In other words, the tryptamine cocktail is likely somewhat similar across most cultivated cubes. Except for a few unique strains that have been interbred for higher psilocybin concentrations, the old adage of 'cubes are cubes' held strong.

THE STORY OF SUBS

Things got a little more interesting in McTaggart's work when he genetically analysed a more local species of mushroom – subs.

Psychedelically inclined mushroom hunters in the southern states of Australia are likely to be familiar with the local 'shroom season' – that stretch of a few months, starting late in autumn, when a very particular species of magic mushroom appears almost everywhere. This is *Psilocybe subaeruginosa*.

Unlike mushroom foragers in northern Australian states, who hunt by covertly sneaking around cow pastures looking for cubes in slops of animal dung, sub hunters are more local, more urban and, dare I say it, maybe more sophisticated. After all, sub hunters aren't digging through literal shit for their magic mushrooms.

Subs are wood-loving mushrooms and their favourite habitat is pine bark, the very same material that happens to be a landscaping staple in every local park and playground in metropolitan regions. Come shroom season, Aussie sub hunters head to their local parks and often find exactly what they're looking for.

What most magic-mushroom hunters in the southern states of Australia probably don't realise is that their local subs are unique magic mushrooms. For one, they are old. Really old.*

As we learned earlier, psilocybin mushrooms first emerged around 66 million years ago as fungi that inhabit decomposing plant matter. Then, around 57 million years ago, there was an evolutionary split into two separate paths. From here, magic mushrooms found homes in a variety of ecological niches, attaching their mycelial networks to decomposing wood before figuring out ways to grow directly in soil. Some species then shifted to finding transitory homes in animal dung.

Questions around the origins of different magic-mushroom species are a hot topic in mycology circles. McTaggart wanted to find out where subs come from. The fun of genetic studies can be in tracing a species back to its earliest geographical location.

The issue with Aussie subs, you see, is they look very similar to two North American species of psilocybes: *P. azurescens* and *P. cyanescens*.[23] And can you imagine how defensive psychonauts in the Northern Hemisphere could be to certain questions about the origins of their magic mushrooms?

McTaggart's findings landed like a nuclear bomb in the world of mycology nerds.[24] By tracing the genomes of more than 80 samples gathered from all over the east coast of Australia, McTaggart comprehensively showed that *P. azurescens* and *P. cyanescens* in the Northern Hemisphere were genetically the same species as *P. subaeruginosa*. And not only that, but those Northern Hemisphere mushrooms seemed to have only relatively recently infiltrated ecosystems in both the Americas and Europe.

* There is some semantic debate around calling subs an 'old' species. Like every other species, subs have continually evolved over time so it's fair to say calling a species 'old' isn't exactly an accurate way to describe something. Caine Barlow suggests the most diplomatic way to put it would be to say subs are 'a modern version of something likely to be very, very old'.

His findings provocatively suggested Australia was probably the home of wood-loving magic mushrooms, and that it was likely only in the last few hundred years that this species invaded the Northern Hemisphere. American mycologists weren't happy with this conclusion.

This wasn't the only unexpected finding in McTaggart's studies. He also zoomed in on the psilocybin gene cluster and saw something really strange.

Every *P. subaeruginosa* sample contained an unusual gene duplication feature. The species seemed to consistently carry three versions of the PsiH gene – one of the genes that codes for an enzyme crucial to the creation of psilocybin. One of those extra PsiH genes was non-functional in all samples, according to McTaggart. But the third wasn't. In fact, in around 30 per cent of samples he tested, this additional PsiH gene was active.

McTaggart suggests there must be some evolutionarily beneficial reason for *P. subaeruginosa* to have conserved this feature. It's doing something ... but what?

'It's like having a duplication of a gene and then that gene, that new copy, has the freedom to explore,' McTaggart explains, after I ask to have this slightly complicated bit of science dumbed down. 'And if it doesn't give an evolutionary disadvantage ... then it'll stick around. And then if it gives an advantage, it'll end up just becoming fixed, like, "Okay, we really benefit from this gene being here. So you're in, mate." And with subs, there's been these two gene duplications.'

McTaggart's findings with magic-mushroom genetic diversity led to a thought-provoking conclusion. Could some magic mushrooms be generating significantly novel combinations of tryptamines? And could these tryptamines, other than psilocybin and psilocin, be affecting the nature of a psychedelic experience?

For years psychonauts have come up with elaborate ways to describe different psychedelic experiences when comparing various magic mushrooms. Some shrooms give more internal trips. Some are heavy, some are light. Some are more social, while others throw you down on the couch.

For the most part, scientists have presumed those differing descriptions were merely the result of stronger or weaker doses of psilocybin/psilocin combined with the specificity of a person's mindset and environment during a trip: dose, set and setting. But McTaggart's research gestured to something else. Could the cocktail of different tryptamines in a given magic mushroom influence the 'taste' of the trip?

THE ENTOURAGE EFFECT

Back in 1998, a small study was published in the *European Journal of Pharmacology*.[25] It was an unpretentious and rather niche piece of research looking at how the activity of certain psychoactive molecules could be amplified by a couple of other naturally occurring molecules that were, by themselves, pharmacologically inactive.

From this small study, the idea of the 'entourage effect' was birthed. In simple terms the hypothesis suggests it is possible the biological effect of certain natural products, from either plants or animals, can be potentiated or amplified through a synergy with other compounds present in their original context. By themselves these other molecules may not do much, but in combination they work together to do quite a lot.

Most entourage-effect research is concentrated around cannabis, and it's fair to say there is still great debate over whether it is real or not. For every bit of positive research on the subject[26] you can find another study countering the existence of the phenomenon. In fact, a thorough scoping review on the topic, published in 2023, suggested the current literature on the entourage effect in cannabis to be 'contradictory, equivocal, and inconclusive ... with both advocates and critics of the "entourage effect" expressing their observations and opinions in several reviews, based primarily on the same existing original articles, of which there are relatively few'.[27]

With the entourage effect already a contentious subject in the scientific world,[28] we turn back to the world of psilocybin.

McTaggart believes the current field of psychedelic science operates from a profoundly narrow perspective. In his view there is a dominant but frustratingly reductive view that the pharmacological action of psychedelics comes down to just one set of receptors in the brain.

'The dogma is that in a psilocybin experience, all that matters is psilocin binding to 5-HT2A receptors. And that's it!' McTaggart explains in a kind of exasperated tone. He says most subjective variations and therapeutic outcomes are thought to be related to environmental factors – the classic 'set and setting' idea – and how much psilocybin you consume. But, he asks, what if these other molecules are doing something?

'I think it's better to keep an open mind, especially when we don't even understand how it's working! When there's this whole other suite of compounds there, it seems a bit premature to be so dogmatic.'

So what do we know about these other compounds in magic mushrooms?

Surprisingly little, as it turns out.

THE CURIOUS CASE OF AERUGINASCIN

After completing their landmark survey into cases of mushroom-induced paralysis, Simon Beck and Caine Barlow were confident wood-lover paralysis was real. It had affected too many people, in too many disparate conditions, to be just an artifact of the trip. The next step was to figure out what could be in certain kinds of magic mushrooms to cause this phenomenon.

Beck remembered coming across a random post by a researcher named Barbara Bauer, on a website called *Psychedelic Science Review*. The short article, published in 2019, presented a novel explanation for the phenomenon of wood-lover paralysis. Dubbed 'The Aeruginascin Hypothesis', Bauer speculated that the tryptamine aeruginascin, very rarely detected in some psilocybin mushrooms, could be responsible for the paralytic condition.[29]

To get to grips with Bauer's hypothesis, lets take a closer look at our psilocybin biosynthesis path.

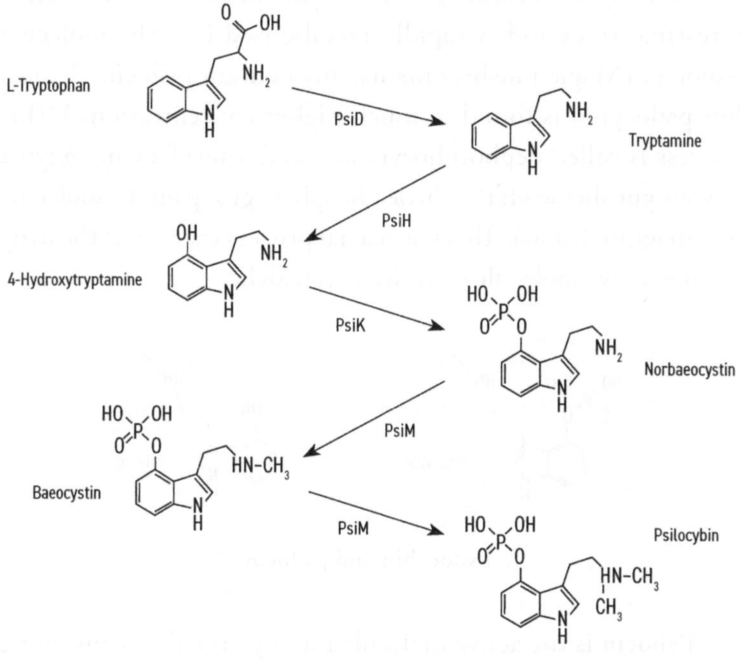

The synthesis of psilocybin from the amino acid tryptophan

As we look at the chain of events a molecule goes through when a mushroom synthesises psilocybin from tryptophan, at the end of the process we see the job of the PsiM gene is to add a little arm to the branch on the right of the molecule. This is called 'adding a methyl group', and the final result, psilocybin, shares a resemblance to one of the common neurotransmitters in our bodies: serotonin (below).

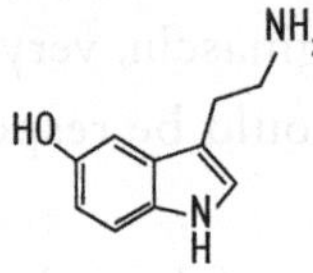

Serotonin

When you consume psilocybin, the drug hits your gastrointestinal tract and is rapidly metabolised into the molecule psilocin. (Magic mushrooms usually contain psilocin already, but psilocybin is found in much higher concentrations.) This process is called dephosphorylation, and it involves an enzyme in your gut slicing off that little phosphate group on the molecule (see diagram below). This is a crucial process that turns the drug from inactive molecule to active psychedelic.

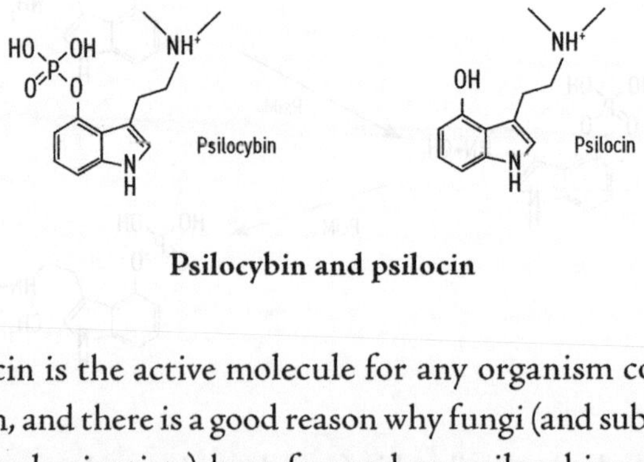

Psilocybin and psilocin

Psilocin is the active molecule for any organism consuming psilocybin, and there is a good reason why fungi (and subsequently our medical scientists) have focused on psilocybin: psilocin is notoriously unstable. It degrades easily in the presence of light and oxygen; even synthesised psilocin is a challenging molecule to make and keep active. Psilocybin is the much safer, stable molecule to produce, even though it isn't really in the ultimate form it needs to be to get into those key serotonin receptors. For almost all organisms that consume psilocybin, this is not a problem. We just eat up the psilocybin, transform it in our gut, and bingo, get equal amounts of psilocin.

We see psilocybin has two little branches, called methyl groups (bold text in the diagram below), but what happens if somehow a third little branch appears?

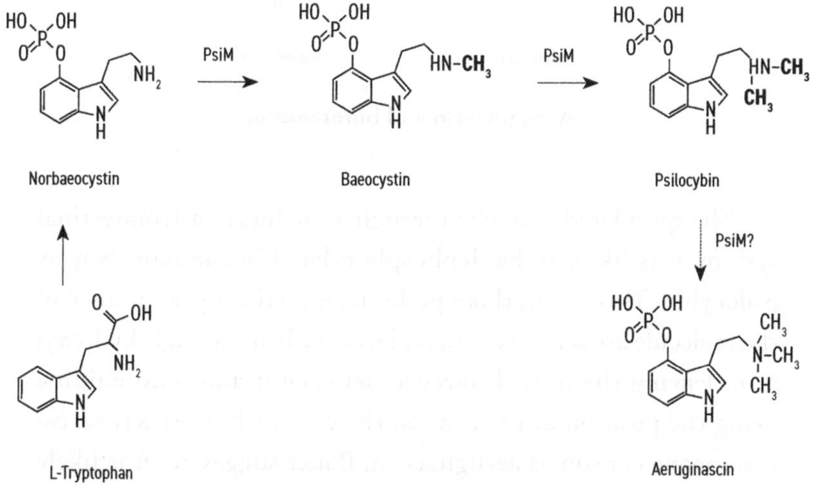

The synthesis of aeruginascin

This leaves us with a molecule called aeruginascin, a tryptamine that has been found in some species of psilocybe mushrooms.[30]

What does aeruginascin do? We don't really know. It was only discovered in 1989 when a mycologist was studying compounds found in a European mushroom called *Inocybe aeruginascens*.

At the time, the researcher hypothesised the molecule could modify the action of psilocybin in some kind of psychedelic entourage effect, creating a more euphoric experience. This conclusion was based on the researcher's own anecdotal observations.[31]

Barbara Bauer, on the other hand, presented a very different suggestion for what aeruginascin could do when consumed by a human. Bauer noted the aeruginascin molecule was incredibly similar to another molecule known as bufotenidine.

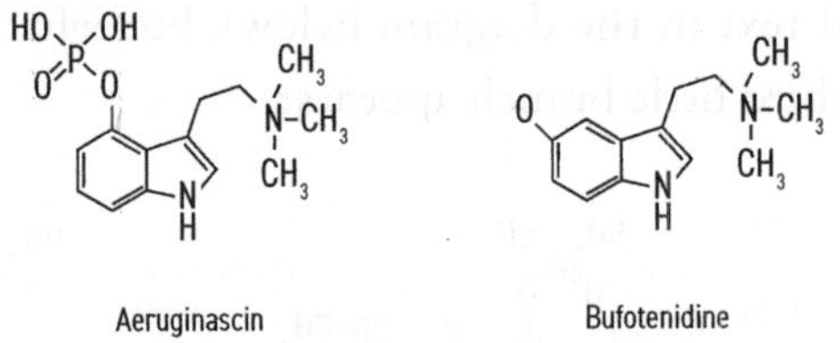

Aeruginascin and bufotenidine

She speculated that when aeruginascin hits a gastrointestinal system, it is likely to be dephosphorylated in the same way as psilocybin. This means those pesky arms on the top left branch of the molecule are removed and replaced with just a single hydroxyl arm, leaving the only difference between it and bufotenidine being the position of the arm on the core carbon structure. So if someone consumes aeruginascin, Bauer suggested, it is likely metabolised into a molecule very similar to bufotenidine.

Bufotenidine is a known toxin found in toad venom. Research is relatively scarce on the molecule, but there were some early mouse studies in the 1970s that found it acted as a paralytic agent. The interesting thing is that, despite bufotenidine sharing some similarities with serotonin and psilocybin, that third arm on the big branch actually keeps the molecule from being able to cross the blood–brain barrier – meaning that bufotenidine, and likely aeruginascin, mostly exert effects on the peripheral nervous system and not the brain. It is this idea that underpinned Bauer's aeruginascin hypothesis for wood-lover paralysis. Could unusually high levels of aeruginascin be causing the strange paralytic effects?

Simon Beck started digging further into this idea. His observations on how wood-lover paralysis presents in humans led him to diverge slightly from Bauer's initial hypothesis. Bauer suggested the paralytic mechanism of aeruginascin came about through the molecule's interaction with 5-HT3 receptors. These are part of the body's serotonin system and 5-HT3 receptors can be found all over the human body.

But Beck felt like something else was going on. His survey into wood-lover paralysis revealed a common trait: the muscle weakness came and went in strange waves. And the more a person worked their muscles, the worse the weakness got – just like Kay's experience the fateful night Rachael Dixon died.

'That's very, very similar to [a condition called] myasthenia gravis, in terms of the way it presents,' Beck told me. Myasthenia gravis is a rare autoimmune disease that displays in muscle weakness, primarily around the face. The weakness occurs because immune system antibodies destroy particular receptors that sit in between the nerve and the muscle. Some animal studies have shown that bufotenindine blocks that same neuromuscular receptor.

When Beck compared the dephosphorylated form of aeruginascin to some commonly used muscle relaxation drugs used in anaesthesia, he saw striking similarities. His current hypothesis is that aeruginascin works as a neuromuscular blocking agent. And *this* is what he thinks causes wood-lover paralysis.

But the proposition raises a whole host of questions. How are magic mushrooms producing aeruginascin? Why do certain mushrooms produce high volumes of aeruginascin and others from the same species don't? Why might mushrooms be producing that compound? And what else could possibly be causing wood-lover paralysis if not aeruginascin?

A NEW TRYPTAMINE?

All of these questions bring us back to McTaggart's work investigating the genetic diversity in the psilocybin gene cluster.

McTaggart's big-picture thesis is the idea that over the course of 66 million years, psilocybe mushrooms infiltrated a variety of different ecological niches. And each time it entered a different environment, the mushroom optimised its tryptamine cocktail for whatever organisms it encountered. This can be detected in the psilocybin gene cluster diversity McTaggart encountered with his studies in subs.

McTaggart isn't particularly convinced by the aeruginascin hypothesis. According to him, there is some research showing the molecule doesn't bind well to 5-HT receptors. He thinks something else is going on in mushrooms to cause the mysterious condition. And the unique thing he discovered with subs is that strange duplication of certain genes in its psilocybin gene cluster.

Why do subs have three iterations of the PsiH gene? One of the two extra genes may be inactive, but what is that active one doing?

McTaggart offers up his wildest speculation: wood-lover paralysis is caused by a novel tryptamine produced in some mushrooms, and we simply haven't identified it yet. He believes that extra active PsiH gene could be doing something strange during the psilocybin biosynthesis process, leading to the production of a new tryptamine – a new drug.

Here, McTaggart's hypothesis somewhat starts to echo Beck's ideas. Underpinning both speculations is the belief that some kind of novel molecule is being produced and it targets a group of peripheral serotonin receptors outside of the brain that control motor function. As McTaggart is clear to point out, we have more than a dozen different serotonin receptors in our bodies, and we know psilocybin binds to more than just one receptor. So what are these other molecules in mushrooms doing?

At the most extreme end of the spectrum we have the example of wood-lover paralysis, but a nightmarish paralytic experience isn't the only thing other tryptamines in magic mushrooms may be doing. One of the more exciting discoveries in recent years has been the work around a molecule in psilocybe mushrooms called norpsilocin.

AN ANTIDEPRESSANT IN MUSHROOMS?

Norpsilocin was only discovered recently, in 2017, after a trio of microbiologists in Germany stumbled across it while poking around *P. cubensis* mushrooms using high-resolution mass spectrometry.[32] In the same way psilocin is a dephosphorylated form of psilocybin, it was speculated that this newly characterised molecule was a dephosphorylated form of baeocystin.

We don't really know what norpsilocin does to a human brain but early preclinical experiments have proved fascinating. One 2024 study by a team of psychologists and pharmacologists in the United States looked at the biological and behavioural effects of several mushroom tryptamines, including norpsilocin and aeruginascin.[33] The study confirmed that aeruginascin, in its dephosphorylated form (known as 4-hydroxy-*N,N,N*-trimethyl-tryptamine or 4-HO-TMT), cannot cross the blood–brain barrier. The study also found that both norpsilocin and 4-hydroxy-tryptamine (4-HT) – the dephosphorylated form of norbaeocystin – could bind with 5-HT2A receptors as well as psilocin.

We now know psilocybin isn't the only mushroom tryptamine that gets into our brain and goes for those crucial serotonin receptors. But things get a little more exciting when we look at the other data from this landmark study.

In trying to understand what kind of behavioural effects are produced by norpsilocin and 4-HT, the researchers looked to a pair of classic rodent behaviour experiments. The first was what is known as the head-twitch response.

Studying psychedelics in animals is difficult, to say the least. Scientists can't exactly give a drug to a mouse and ask it whether it's having a mystical psychedelic experience. The only test we currently have to give us a clue about whether a drug can generate psychedelic-like effects in animals is the head-twitch response.

It was first described back in the 1950s when scientists were experimenting with LSD.[34] Rats given moderate doses of a psychedelic were seen to produce a curious head-shake behaviour – something akin to the way a wet dog shakes its body dry. It took a couple of decades for scientists to understand this head-twitch response could serve as an effective predictor for psychedelic effects in humans.

To put it simply: you give a rodent a drug that stimulates its 5-HT2A receptors and it will shake its head in a very recognisable way.[35] Therefore it was generally assumed any drug that effectively stimulates 5-HT2A receptors will cause psychedelic-like effects in humans. However, more recently, scientists have blown that assumption up by developing novel molecules targeting that receptor with no hallucinogenic effects. At least we *think* that's the case when these novel drugs are tested using the head-twitch response in rodents – to date, almost all these supposedly non-hallucinogenic 5-HT2A agonists have yet to be tested in humans. What kinds of subjective effects they actually generate is still unknown.

The recent study looking into norpsilocin and 4-HT was the first to reveal that these two tryptamines naturally found in magic mushrooms do not generate any head-twitch response in rodents. While they seemed to hit 5-HT2A receptors as powerfully as psilocin, they didn't appear to generate the psychedelic effects we would expect.

Things got even stranger when looking at the results of the next test.

Just as challenging as knowing whether an animal is tripping on a psychedelic is knowing whether an animal is deeply depressed. One commonly used experiment to test the efficacy of an antidepressant drug is a controversial practice called the 'forced swimming test', which involves dropping a rodent in a cylinder filled with water. In the late 1970s, researchers discovered rodents tended to vigorously swim for a short amount of time before shifting to a relatively immobile position, using minimal movement to keep their nose above water. The test was initially called the 'behavioural despair test' as it was thought to measure an animal's sense of hopelessness. When antidepressant drugs such as selective serotonin reuptake inhibitors (SSRIs) were given to the rodents, their swimming behaviours tended to last much longer than they did without medication. Over time scientists suggested the test was a somewhat accurate measure for negative mood and the subsequent efficacy of mood-modifying medicines.

In recent years the test has been criticised for both its inaccuracy and its cruelty to animals. A review in the early 2000s found the test proved reliable as a screening tool for antidepressant drugs but many researchers recently began moving away from its use.[36] In 2024, the state of New South Wales became the first region in the world to outright ban the use of the test.

However, this research team in the US used the forced swimming test to compare the effects of psilocin with 4-HT, norpsilocin, and a common antidepressant called fluoxetine. While we already knew psilocin generated antidepressant effects in rats, the study surprisingly discovered norpsilocin to have similar effects to psilocin and the common antidepressant fluoxetine. Despite questions over the accuracy of the test, it offers a compelling clue to the effects of norpsilocin.

The headline here is that norpsilocin doesn't generate psychedelic effects, but it may confer antidepressant properties.

'I DIDN'T GET HIGH'

Here we return to McTaggart's exciting and strange idea. He steadfastly doesn't believe psilocybin (or, more specifically, psilocin) is all that matters in a magic-mushroom experience – both from a therapeutic and phenomenological outcome.

'I would say that we have enough information to reject the hypothesis that it's only psilocin binding to 5-HT2A receptors when you eat a whole mushroom. And that's because you've got two other tryptamines that are competing for space at serotonin receptors. So to say that that doesn't impact an experience I think needs further testing.'

But things get a little more wild in this new world of magic-mushroom science. Could certain combinations of tryptamines make some mushrooms more effective at, say, treating depression, compared to just psilocybin by itself? Could a mushroom with a subjectively 'heavy' body trip be carrying small amounts of tryptamines that are directly affecting the peripheral nervous system?

'Maybe, I don't know – this is now speculation,' McTaggart cautiously adds. 'Maybe if you've taken a mushroom that has a high concentration or a high ratio of norpsilocin to psilocin, maybe something else is happening in your head compared to just taking pure psilocin and that's because you've got something that has an antidepressant activity competing for space at your serotonin receptors.'

Just like psilocin is the tryptamine that psilocybin turns into when it enters an organism, norpsilocin comes from its parent molecule baeocystin. At the time of writing this book, we have virtually no knowledge of what baeocystin (or norpsilocin) does in humans. But, like many pharmacological mysteries, there are some psychonaut chemists out there doing self-experiments.

In 2019, mycologist Paul Stamets appeared on the Joe Rogan podcast to discuss a few mushroom-related topics.[37] One of the weirder conversational tangents emerged when Stamets started talking about baeocystin. He recounted an experience where he obtained some pure baeocystin to try. He set up the story by explaining the context surrounding his experiment. It was a period of relatively high anxiety for Stamets after a large and expensive research trip to Antarctica had just been unexpectedly cancelled at the last minute.

It was in this mood that he sat down, with a doctor friend monitoring his vital signs, and took 10 milligrams of pure baeocystin. Ten minutes passed – nothing. Twenty minutes – nothing. The doctor checked Stamets' vital signs and it seemed like there were mild signs of a drug-like effect – for example, his pupils had dilated – so something had hit some serotonin receptors in his brain. But he definitely wasn't high or having anything akin to a psychedelic experience.

'I didn't get high,' Stamets recounted on the podcast in 2019. 'She [the doctor] goes, "How do you feel?" And I said, "I feel great! I have no anxiety. Everything with this trip is going to be fine."'

Stamets believes baeocystin potentially has a profound anti-anxiety effect but, of course, this is just one man and one random, isolated self-experiment.

A massive question often raised when scientists on the fringe of things start talking about the effects of secondary tryptamines in magic mushrooms is that all these other compounds have only ever been detected in extraordinarily low concentrations. When tryptamines are generally measured in magic mushrooms, it is primarily psilocybin seen in any relevant concentration. If I was taking, say, 3 or 4 grams of dried magic mushrooms, I could expect to be consuming anywhere from 15 to 25 milligrams of psilocybin. This is analogous to the dose of pure psilocybin used in clinical research. Alongside that volume of psilocybin, the levels of other tryptamines are considered negligible. Barely 1–2 milligrams of baeocystin can be detected in that same volume of magic mushrooms.

But McTaggart's chemical research uncovered something surprising. He discovered the most common method researchers use to extract psilocybin from magic mushrooms is likely to degrade other tryptamines. So many of the tryptamine ratios we have previously tracked in mushrooms could be fundamentally wrong.

'All of those [mushroom] extracts are usually extracted in methanol or an alcohol,' McTaggart explains. 'And from what we've found with our preliminary work, the solvent makes a difference. So norpsilocin and 4-HT are less soluble in alcohols than psilocybin. You're automatically measuring a lower ratio of them.'

Not only that, but in 2025 a few studies started to suggest that norpsilocin and 4-HT are possibly better at binding to 5-HT2A receptors than the psychedelic psilocin. This means, in some mushrooms, you probably have a few milligrams of other tryptamines, and these molecules are beating psilocin to the 5-HT2A receptors. What might they be doing?

'What if you've got a 100 per cent binding rate of the small amount of norpsilocin there compared to psilocin?' McTaggart exclaims, in what I was starting to see as a characteristic kind of enthused exasperation. 'What's it doing at the receptor? We don't know.'

DESIGNER MAGIC MUSHROOMS

And here we are. Left with a bunch of lingering questions.

The story of wood-lover paralysis is still incomplete. It was only in mid-2025 that the very first academic article on the phenomenon was published.[38] Co-authored by Simon Beck and Caine Barlow, alongside researchers Liam Engel and Monica Barratt, the article filled a longstanding hole in the literature, offering the first valid, published resource for scientists to point to and say, 'Yes, this is a real thing.'

But science is slow sometimes. And the mystery of what is causing the paralysis remains. In our last conversation, McTaggart tells me there are finally a few samples of mushrooms known to cause the paralysis being tested in a couple of labs around Australia. All he can tell me at this point is that tryptamine levels in the samples tested were 'off the charts'. There seems to be some unknown molecules in the samples that have yet to be formally characterised.

In late July 2025, the Victorian coroner released a long-awaited report on the death of Rachael Dixon. The cause of death was labelled 'unascertained'. There was no pathological explanation as to why Rachael passed away that night. No sign of heart disease. No biomarkers of seizure or inflammation.

Accompanying the coroner's report was a lengthy set of comments mostly detailing communications with Simon Beck about the phenomenon of wood-lover paralysis. The coroner expressed gratitude for being made aware of this little-known phenomenon, and agreed the scenario appeared consistent with the condition. But that's as far as the coroner took it, admitting in the report that 'without a confirmed mechanism [that can be] ascertained forensically, I ultimately determined on the balance of probabilities that I am unable to find wood-lover paralysis caused or contributed to Rachael's death'.

It's a sad question mark to leave the report on, but it is the first time the phenomenon has been formally cited in a public coroner's report. And the report concludes with the coroner citing Beck's study, in an indirect way of getting the word out to help prevent future harm:

> Information about WLP [wood-lover paralysis] should be included in education about psilocybin mushrooms, both for consumers and service providers. Growing awareness of WLP effects, which mushrooms are most likely to produce WLP and syndrome management strategies for consumers and carers (e.g. avoid physical tasks, ensure temperature control, etc.) can help control this growing risk and should inform how markets are regulated.[39]

I was left with a few wild questions. Can we make designer psychedelic mushrooms by genetically tweaking the tryptamine make-up? Can we develop customised tryptamine cocktails to generate more colourful visual trip experiences? Maybe generate a feeling that someone is light on their feet? Or how about other trips that are heavier, slower, less colourful but more restful? Or could we even produce mushrooms that are explicitly for depression or anxiety, with less subjective psychedelia and more antidepressant actions? Therapy shrooms?

McTaggart thinks this is all entirely possible but he's sceptical we'll be getting anywhere close to this reality any time soon. You see, modern medical science is often dogmatic and pharmaceutical research isn't exploratory.

The paradigm is often galvanised into one lane. We focus on a single chemical molecule. Highlight its properties. Study its effects in a focused and controlled way. Conduct placebo or dose-controlled trials to tell us what that drug does. Then give pure and predictable doses to people suffering from particular medical conditions.

This system has served us well for many decades. It has produced a magnificent array of life-saving medicines. But what if this kind of process doesn't particularly suit magic mushrooms? Who is going to run an elaborate clinical trial testing different combinations of pure psilocybin with baeocystin or 4-HT? How about spiking psilocybin with some norpsilocin for a better antidepressant result?

All of these questions don't come close to the even harder problem of tinkering with the phenomenological effects of a trip. Can we customise the subjective properties of a psychedelic trip? Can we make a trip less 'trippy'? And if we can, what does that mean for the overall experience?

Some researchers think we can do this. But in the meantime, Alistair McTaggart is hoping broader decriminalisation policies will help unlock his world of designer magic-mushroom research. He thinks it is much more likely we'll only ever truly understand how these different tryptamine cocktails work by getting a bunch of brash psychonauts together to legally test new breeds of magic mushrooms.

This is the real final frontier for consciousness exploration: engineering the psilocybin gene cluster in magic mushrooms to create novel psychedelic experiences.

And, as usual, we humans are only just catching up with a game nature has already been playing for millions of years.

3

MICRODOSING

HOW TO DESIGN A CLINICAL TRIAL

'You took too much, man! You took too much!'

Dr Gonzo (Benicio del Toro), in the film
Fear and Loathing in Las Vegas, 1998

Turn on, tune in and drop out.

The infamous refrain from Timothy Leary in the 1960s succinctly encapsulated the psychedelic philosophy of the counterculture. And the first two parts of that aphorism worked just fine for most people.

'Turn on': take the drug, activate your consciousness. 'Tune in': find a harmony or synchronicity with the world around you. But that final step – the 'drop out' part – presented a bit of a threat to the status quo.

In the 1980s, Leary tried to clarify what he meant by dropping out, calling it 'an active, selective, graceful process of detachment from involuntary or unconscious commitments'.[1] At the time it was first proposed, however, it felt more like a clarion call to the youth. The idea that psychedelics were being used as a tool to get a whole generation to drop out of conventional society sent bolts of fear through the establishment: 'We can't have people dropping out of all the systems that hold up our world. We *need* them to keep coming to work. We *need* them to keep paying taxes. We *need* them to keep running on the hamster wheel.'

For much of the second half of the 20th century, psychedelics were intrinsically intertwined with alternative subcultures that were fundamentally opposed to mainstream systems. It was thought psychedelic drugs so deeply deconstructed one's pre-existing beliefs that the 'drop out' part of the process was inevitable.

But what if we could get all the socially functional benefits of psychedelics – energy, creativity, mood boosts – without the pesky mind-altering, life-changing, hallucinogenic experience? What if we could do the 'turn on' and 'tune in' parts but not 'drop out'? Could psychedelics become something akin to strong coffee, so we take the drugs *and* go to work? In fact, what if we take the drugs and work more efficiently?

Welcome to the wonderful world of microdosing psychedelics. You can finally have your cake and eat it too. Feel your anxieties wash away, your clouds of depression lift. Colours are brighter. Everything is just … better.

Microdosing is a perfect symbiosis between Western capitalism and psychedelics. It's also a phenomenon where popular practice has raced ahead of scientific study. There is very little research into whether psychedelic microdosing actually does what its advocates say it does. For all we know, microdosing could be a kind of psychedelic homeopathy, where people take tiny, imperceptible doses of a substance and claim to garner life-changing benefits.

For most of this modern psychedelic renaissance, researchers have been studying high doses of psychedelics, but I wanted to find someone who was thinking small. Luckily enough one of the world's first placebo-controlled microdosing clinical trials was taking place in Sydney. And I went to the home of the trial, Macquarie University, to see just how you figure out whether psychedelic microdosing works.

BEFORE WE GET TO THE TRIAL, IT IS WORTH QUICKLY understanding where microdosing came from, because in many ways it is a distinctly modern phenomenon. There is very little historical precedent to microdosing. Some anthropological evidence suggests low, almost sub-psychoactive doses of mescaline have been tracked in certain traditional preparations, and one study reported the practice of children, or even babies, being given tiny doses of psychedelics in parts of Brazil.[2] However, these reports are rare, and the way modern microdosing is practised (multiple tiny doses each week for several months at a time) is a very Western way of taking drugs or supplements.

If we had to put a pin on the birthdate of psychedelic microdosing, we could probably look to a book published in 2011 called *The Psychedelic Explorer's Guide.*[3] Written by American researcher James Fadiman, the book featured a chapter titled 'Can Sub-Perceptual Doses of Psychedelics Improve Normal Functioning?'

Fadiman first turned on to psychedelics in the early 1960s after a Harvard professor named Richard Alpert (aka Ram Dass) handed him two psilocybin pills at a cafe in Paris. He ended up at Stanford in the heady days of the swinging '60s; living next to Ken Kesey, a foundational counterculture figure who would go on to found the pro-LSD hippy community called the Merry Pranksters. Fadiman studied psychedelics firsthand at Stanford until the big prohibition wave brought everything to a standstill.

Over the following decades Fadiman built a prolific and diverse career blending psychology with Eastern philosophy and psychedelic ideas, until a random conversation in the late 2000s sent him down a novel path. Meeting with a colleague, Fadiman was told that Albert Hofmann, the originator of LSD in the 1940s, had reportedly spoken about the beneficial personal effects of taking very low doses of the psychedelic.

According to Fadiman's recollection, he misheard the dose he was told Hofmann had taken. Fadiman thought he was told Hofmann was taking as little as 10 micrograms of LSD – and this fascinated him. Such a low dose would have been barely perceptible, so Fadiman started up some citizen science research to see what would happen when people took such tiny amounts.

For a few years after *The Psychedelic Explorer's Guide* was published, the practice of microdosing quietly bubbled away in psychonaut circles across the world – quietly heralded as a mild antidepressant. But things changed when a group of tech entrepreneurs embraced the idea, and twentysomething computer guys in Silicon Valley began using low doses of psychedelics as a way to 'biohack' their creativity. Come late 2015, an article in *Rolling Stone* magazine finally catapulted the practice into the mainstream. Journalists from *Forbes*, *Wired* and other magazines quickly followed; everyone was jockeying to publish a psychedelic microdosing story.[4] 'It's like tuning a guitar,' one evangelical user suggested. 'It helps me think more creatively,' another white-collar San Francisco worker declared.[5]

By 2016 psychedelic microdosing was the hip new thing to do. It worked, apparently, although not one researcher had actually studied the anecdotal phenomenon.

'I WANTED TO KNOW: IS THIS REAL OR IS IT PLACEBO?'

Vince Polito was nearing the end of his undergraduate degree in psychology when a friend invited him to a sweat lodge ceremony – a traditional purification ritual that originated in Central America. The idea is that one spends an extended period of time in a super-heated hut, triggering a kind of altered state of consciousness from the sweltering surrounds. Open to new experiences, Polito went along, not really knowing what the whole thing was about. After several hours inside a hut that was steamy, dark and stiflingly hot, Polito emerged exhausted but, strangely, feeling good.

For this budding researcher the experience was fascinating: physically challenging but equally invigorating. He particularly enjoyed the communal nature of the ceremony and, as he started chatting with other participants outside, he began to hear remarkable stories of people having hallucinatory visions and out-of-body experiences. 'I hadn't had anything like that happen,' Polito told me.

> And I was just fascinated. Were these true reports? Did people really have those experiences? If they did, how come I didn't have an experience like that? If that's not a true report, then what's making the person feel like that's what they should be saying in this context? I was just immediately fascinated by these interrelated kinds of questions. What are the mechanisms of consciousness change? What's the social context that shapes the way that people interpret the experiences that they have?

Polito's psychology honours project ended up immersed in this unique world of sweat lodges. He surveyed scores of participants, trying to identify what kinds of pre-existing beliefs and emotional states led to someone being more likely to have an altered-consciousness experience. What were the factors that primed someone to be susceptible to an out-of-body experience?

Moving into his PhD, Polito was wary of wading too far into the fringes of consciousness research. After all, it was the early 2000s, and altered-states studies were still relatively taboo. There wasn't an academic path for 'weird' research. But he found common ground with some other academics who were looking into the way highly hypnotisable people lose a sense of agency over their actions when they are hypnotised. The phenomenon of hypnosis was another perfect example of how expectation and influence can lead to big shifts in a person's consciousness. Not everyone could be effectively hypnotised, just in the same way not everyone came out of a sweat lodge with stories of hallucinatory visions.

By 2016 Polito was well and truly done with his PhD and working as a research fellow at Macquarie University. His group was mostly focused on how unusual beliefs form in certain communities, and how placebo and expectation can fuel powerful movements. At the same time, stories about psychedelic microdosing were all over the news. So Polito finally leaped at the opportunity he had been waiting years for. He was perfectly poised to be one of the first researchers in the world to seriously study the phenomenon of microdosing.

'I wanted to know: is this real or is it placebo? So I just took the plunge into doing something on psychedelics. And the first thing we did was an observational study where we found people already microdosing, tracked them for six weeks, and saw what differences they reported from baseline.'

Across 12 months, up to April 2017, Polito and colleague Richard Stevenson tracked nearly 100 microdosers. Alongside requesting brief daily ratings of feelings like connectedness, creativity and wellbeing, the researchers gathered a battery of data at the start and end of the six-week survey.

Ultimately published in early 2019, the study was one of the very first robust investigations into the practice of microdosing, and it delivered some unexpected results.[6] The daily dosing data unsurprisingly revealed reports of improved focus and productivity for about 24 hours after taking a microdose, but the longitudinal data told a different story.

At the end of the six-week study, the researchers found microdosers did report clear improvements in a few key areas. Mental health markers were better, with reduced rates of depression and stress. Significant reductions in the trait of mind-wandering was also seen in the cohort, suggesting some subjective benefits in their capacity to focus on a task.

However, a large number of traits tracked in the study were unchanged after six weeks of microdosing, including reports of overall quality of life, creativity and mindfulness. On top of this, the data suggested the microdosers demonstrated a small increase in neurotic traits.

Polito and Stevenson were surprised by this initial data, so they ran a second part to the study. Keeping prior recruitment channels open, they switched the survey from collecting microdosing reports to tracking microdosing expectations. The duo essentially wanted to know whether one's general expectations surrounding what they think microdosing will do sync up with the results of what microdosing is actually doing.

Here, the conclusions were even more intriguing. The things most people expected microdosing to improve – wellbeing, mindfulness and creativity – were the things that were unchanged. The overall takeaway from this landmark bit of research was that psychedelic microdosing is not necessarily doing nothing, but it also doesn't seem to be doing what people *expect* it to do.

For Polito, this was an exciting discovery. He had been working in the field of cognitive psychology, tracking how expectations influence outcomes, for years. It also left him in a strange position, stuck in between two highly polarised camps: one vociferously arguing microdosing is all placebo effect, and the other selling the practice as a cure-all for everything that ails you.

THE 'SELF-BLINDED' STUDY

After that 2019 study was published, a flurry of microdosing research started appearing in scientific journals. Finally, researchers were catching up with the popular practice after a few years of it being 'out in the wild'. But these were all still observational investigations in people microdosing at home.

There was imprecision to this type of naturalistic research. Doses were randomly eyeballed by psychonauts guessing how much LSD was on the blotters they were soaking, or how much psilocybin was in the mushrooms they were grinding up. The entire practice was also a bit of a self-fulfilling phenomenon. The people who were microdosing obviously did it because they had expectations it would be beneficial, and they only continued to do it if they felt it was working. So most people taking part in observational microdosing studies would, of course, report it as being positive. Why else would they be doing it?

Around that same time a team of researchers at Imperial College London came up with a magnificent concept for a microdosing study. Since no one at the time was able to get a pure-drug, placebo-controlled clinical trial going, the researchers developed what they called a 'self-blinding' process. The system involved finding people who were microdosing at home and sending them a special kit designed to help them create their own blinded collection of active and placebo doses.

The kit contained several empty opaque capsules. The volunteers would fill a few capsules with their microdose of choice and leave the same amount empty. The capsules were then put into envelopes marked by the researchers with QR codes. The microdoses went into one set of envelopes and the placebos into another set. Only the researchers knew which QR codes were linked to active doses and which were placebos. The volunteers shuffled their envelopes and then randomly drew one each week for four weeks, not knowing what was in any given week's collection of doses.

It was a remarkably clever design for a trial; the researchers had found a way to get some placebo control into naturalistic drug use. And the results, published in early 2021, were equally fascinating.[7] The big takeaway was that the researchers saw no major differences between microdose weeks and placebo weeks on all the psychological measures they were tracking.

That's not to say people didn't improve across the stretch of the study. Improvements were tracked across a whole host of scales – from mood and energy to creativity – but most interestingly the biggest predictor of improvement wasn't *what* the participants had taken in a given week, but what the participants *thought* they had taken. So, regardless of whether they'd got a microdose or not, if they thought they'd got a microdose, then they tended to show greater improvements across all measures compared to when they thought they'd got a placebo.

Polito was fascinated by that kind of trial design. In lieu of getting a more rigorous investigation off the ground, he adapted the self-blinding microdose model into a neuroimaging experiment. Across 2021 and 2022, Polito recruited around 40 volunteers who microdosed either LSD or magic mushrooms. He developed a simple kit to send participants, allowing them to make one genuine microdose and one placebo. Like the London study, the participants wouldn't know which dose was which.

Each subject came into Polito's lab twice, on the days they were to take either their microdose or placebo. They completed a barrage of tests but the biggest focus was completing a magnetoencephalography (MEG) scan. This is a relatively sophisticated neuroimaging technology designed to track the way different regions of the brain are communicating with one another.

The self-blinding study served as a stepping stone to Polito's current clinical trial: the first big, robust, placebo-controlled investigation into psilocybin microdosing.

The trial was conceived during the claustrophobic early days of the pandemic. Alongside the rolling lockdowns, Polito was on parental leave after having his first child. All he could do was sit at home and dream up crazy ideas – so why not see if he could put together a protocol for the world's first psilocybin microdosing trial? But what exactly would a psilocybin microdosing clinical trial look like?

AS I WALKED THROUGH THE LEAFY CAMPUS OF Macquarie University in early 2025, it dawned on me that this was the first time I'd ever visited the site of an ongoing clinical trial. For almost a decade I'd reported on scientific advances, chatted with researchers and dived deep into journal articles. But across that whole time, my engagement with the real process of doing research had been fleeting. Like many journalists, I'd pay attention to a new finding or study as it emerged, and then just move onto the next thing. In some rare cases I'd spend a few weeks thinking and reading about a particular topic, but for most stories the extent of my focus would be the minutes spent reading a press release or a journal article: years of work, by scores of people, reduced to a passing few seconds of someone reading a pithy 'this trial found yada yada yada'.

Of course, for good or ill, this is the nature of modern science. The firehose of new research inevitably gets funnelled into bite-size morsels that are, for many scientists, infuriatingly reductive. But with this particular microdosing clinical trial, I saw an opportunity to really understand the hard work that goes into discovering new knowledge. The novelty and scale of the trial was unlike anything done before so I had to see for myself what went into pulling off a large, modern clinical trial.

Macquarie University is a little different to other higher education institutions in Australia. It's the first, and only, university in the country to fully incorporate a private teaching hospital onto its campus. And in the basement of that hospital is an entire unit devoted to running clinical trials.

It's a lovely campus, on the outskirts of Sydney, nestled on the edges of some lush bushland – perfect for a psychedelic clinical trial. Except once you get to the research space, it feels very much like a hospital/office environment. Following tiny, printed signs declaring 'MicroDep', you find a tiny unit, much like any other clinical practice room. And here is where the landmark multi-year trial testing psilocybin microdosing is taking place.

To understand how you design a clinical trial for something that hasn't really ever been tested before, you need to go back in time a bit. Psychedelic microdosing is so anecdotal, so amorphous; every single decision you make when building out your protocol is rife with controversy. So let's break it down.

WHAT EVEN IS A MICRODOSE ANYWAY?

The very first question you ask is, 'How much of a dose is a microdose?' Is a microdose something you take and notice absolutely no acute effect? Some believe that if you feel something, you have taken too much. In my early reporting on microdosing, that was always the way I described it. A good microdoser should never know when they are microdosing. But Polito never bought into that idea. His cursory field research saw that plenty of people knew when they were on their 'microdose days'. The whole idea of this being some kind of sub-perceptual treatment was, in reality, a bit of a fiction.

Polito was facing a critical decision. Were the researchers going to shoot for such a low dose that this multi-year, multimillion-dollar trial would end up testing a psychedelic version of homeopathy? Or would they switch their thinking around and consider how 'high' they could go without causing a noticeable impairment in participants' day-to-day life?

Not only was there barely any pharmacological data on the effect of low-dose psilocybin in humans, but real-world psilocybin dosing solely consisted of people grinding up dried magic mushrooms and weighing out small doses. How much actual psilocybin people were consuming was completely unknown.

To figure out a dose, Polito had to work backwards. He knew modern psilocybin clinical trials deployed doses that ranged between 20 and 40 milligrams. He also knew some studies deployed introductory doses of around 15 milligrams. So he knew that much psilocybin was enough to make most people feel like they were tripping.

At the other end of the spectrum, there were a couple of studies looking at how much psilocin ends up in a person's bloodstream after taking very low doses of psilocybin. Here, the data suggested 1- or 2-milligram doses converted to virtually untraceable levels of psilocin. While these may be those perfect 'sub-perceptual' levels of microdosing some advocates refer to, from Polito's perspective they were too low to be useful.

'There was one paper that gave people eight different doses, and then sort of plotted the blood concentration of psilocin at different time points,' Polito explained.[8] 'And it found that at 3 milligrams, there was virtually no psilocin. At 6 milligrams, there was a bit. So that made me think, "Okay, three seems too low; six, just based on how close that's getting to a higher dose, seems too high."'

After much hand-wringing, Polito rolled the dice on 4 milligrams as the dose. He knew this would be an amount that participants would likely 'feel', but that wasn't the main problem. Impairment was the primary concern. Could participants take this dose and go about their daily lives with no problems? Could they still work? Drive? Carry on normal conversations?

Until the study actually kicked off, Polito and the team didn't know whether they had shot too high. The first few patients, cautiously dosed in 2024, revealed they had miraculously struck the sweet spot. No reports emerged of participants feeling overwhelmed or overcome with hallucinatory effects. If any effect was going to be found from microdosing, Polito was sure he had hit a dose high enough that would detect it.

But that led to the next big question in developing the protocol for the trial – a question that has been the bane of all modern psychedelic clinical trials. If participants were taking a dose of a drug that led to noticeable psychoactive effects, then those randomly allocated to the placebo would of course immediately know they were in the dud group. This inability to effectively blind the trial would lead to biased results. The active group will likely overestimate the benefits, knowing they had received the real drug, while the placebo group, disappointed in missing out, would overstate null effects – triggering a scenario known as the 'knowcebo' effect.

Polito knew how powerful the placebo response seemed to be with psychedelic microdosing, and he knew it would be a death knell for his data if the blinding between the two groups evaporated.

'IT'S JUST LIKE A COFFEE'

For well over 200 years scientists have been aware of the placebo effect: that strange phenomenon by which a patient improves after being given either a completely inert drug, or a drug with a psychoactive effect that has nothing to do with the illness in question. We know the placebo effect can be powerful, and in developing standards for the modern clinical trial – what scientists today consider the gold standard for evidence – all external factors that could influence a patient's response to the treatment being tested are minimised.

Believe it or not, human beings are surprisingly optimistic animals. If we are unwell, we *want* to feel better. If we are given a pill and told it will make us feel better, we want it to work. And for some of us, that pill *will* make us feel better, regardless of what's in it. In a clinical trial context, this is called the expectancy effect, and it's a big problem for scientists, particularly in the realm of psychiatric research.

One of the largest ongoing controversies in the world of antidepressant drugs is the massively high placebo response often garnered when they are tested in clinical trials. One meta-study suggested placebo responses in antidepressant trials sit around 30 per cent.[9] This means one in three people in the placebo group generally register a beneficial response from what is ultimately nothing more than a sugar pill. This extraordinarily high placebo response makes it sometimes difficult to ascertain an active drug's effects.

The environment of a psychiatric clinical trial is already heightened before you even throw a psychedelic drug into the mix. Psychedelics are not only easy to spot for participants, but they have been subjected to a flood of celebratory and evangelical media reports over the last few years. How many 'psychedelics are miracle drug' stories have you come across?

The inordinate volume of positive expectancy bias one can encounter in psychedelic clinical research has been amusingly dubbed The Pollan Effect, referring to the bestselling psychedelic pop science book *How to Change Your Mind* by journalist Michael Pollan.[10] The idea is that since the publication of this very popular book in 2018, most people volunteering to take part in a psychedelic clinical trial are arriving with wild expectations. They expect the drugs to really work.

One New Zealand researcher also working to test the veracity of microdosing, Suresh Muthukumaraswamy, is sceptical of most modern psychedelic studies because of this very reason. When I spoke to Suresh a few years ago, he told me he thought most modern psychedelic clinical data is likely overexpressing positive results.[11]

You see, expectancy effects work both ways. Not only is someone who gets a psychedelic drug in a trial primed to think it will work, but someone who gets an inactive placebo will likely be super disappointed. This widens the gap in results between placebo and psychedelic, making it seem like psychedelics are stunningly successful when, in fact, all that may have happened is placebo and knowcebo effects were amplified.

One of my favourite studies from the last few years tried to answer this very question: how powerful are one's expectations when taking a psychedelic drug? To explore this, a research team at McGill University in Canada wondered if they could convince people they were tripping on a psychedelic drug even when they were given a placebo.

The study, dubbed 'Tripping on Nothing', was led by a former-magician-turned-PhD-candidate in psychiatry named Jay Olson.[12] Olson knew the power of influence, so he pulled together all the tricks of the magician trade to set up a scenario that could fool a cohort into thinking they had been given a psychedelic drug.

The researchers created a fictional psychedelic drug called iprocin, designed to make sure any pre-existing notions around the effect of known drugs like LSD or psilocybin couldn't influence the subjects' responses. 'The experimenter explained that iprocin was a fast acting and legal drug similar to psychedelic mushrooms,' the team noted in the study. Its effects would start quickly, participants were told, peaking in one to two hours, then quickly fading.

A room was set up to resemble a party environment, with video projections, ambient music, cushions and snacks. Participants were told the environment was designed to test the effects of psychedelic drugs on creativity in a natural environment. To obscure the fact no actual drugs were being administered, the researchers amplified security procedures to give the impression of serious scientific legitimacy.

The experiment began in the building's lobby when a participant first arrived. Their ID was checked, they were given a wristband and then they were told to wait. While more participants arrived for the study, undercover research assistants pretended to be part of the cohort, talking loudly about how friends had taken part in prior experiments and 'had a blast'.

Once in the test room, researchers wearing white lab coats carefully administered the 'drugs' to each participant. One by one, people were given a pink capsule – prior studies had suggested it was the colour most likely to prime someone to feel stimulant effects. Over the next four hours, the lab-coated researchers wandered in and out of the room, scribbling fictitious notes on clipboards, while undercover assistants (dubbed 'confederates') pretended to be participants in the experiment, expressing strong subjective psychedelic feelings to the test group.

'To make it appear as if the drug was having a physiological effect, one confederate with naturally large pupils told some participants individually, "Your pupils are huge! Are mine like that?"' the researchers explained. 'The room contained no mirrors (nor did the bathroom) or phone cameras for participants to verify this statement, and the dark room with red lights naturally dilated their pupils.'

The results were incredible. Just over 60 per cent of the cohort said they felt some kind of drug effect. Only one in three participants were certain they received a placebo; the rest of the cohort weren't sure. Even about half of those participants with prior psychedelic drug experience felt like they had been given a real psychoactive drug.

The big takeaway was that expectations can powerfully influence how a person responds to psychoactive drugs. And for psychedelic clinical trials, the researchers ardently recommended scientists deploy what are called 'active placebos' in future work. These are placebos that confer some kind of physiological effect, in the hope this will convince people they have been given the active drug.

FROM POLITO'S PERSPECTIVE, THE BEST WAY TO get good data around whether microdosing actually works is to amplify the placebo effect as much as possible. One way he planned to do that was to create a dosing room that heightened any psychological response to the drug. He turned a regular old hospital-like research room into a warm, trippy environment with rugs, low lighting and a psychedelic image or two.

On top of that, he knew he needed to use an active placebo. But what was the best drug to use to 'trick' placebo participants into thinking they'd got the real thing?[13]

Other psychedelic trials in the past had used drugs like niacin as their active placebo. Around half an hour after taking a moderate to high dose of niacin, people tend to feel a flushing sensation across their body. However, as an active placebo in psychedelic research, it has only been mildly effective at convincing patients they've been given the real drug.

More effective in the active placebo world are stimulants. Methylphenidate, commonly known as Ritalin, is often the drug of choice here. If you have never taken Ritalin or psychedelics, then the jittery energy boost of methylphenidate is likely a good way to make you think you got the real psychedelic, especially in the context of a microdosing trial where all participants could be likely to expect was a kind of mild stimulation sensation.

But Vince Polito decided to take his active placebo in a milder direction. He chose a caffeine pill for his placebo group. 'In the end we chose caffeine because it's very safe. It's very easy to access, and people are very unlikely to have a bad reaction to it. But the main reason that we chose caffeine was [that] in anecdotal reports, it's pretty common to see people say that the effect of the microdose was a bit like having a cup of coffee.'

According to Polito, we can think of a microdose as like having that strong cup of coffee early in the morning. Everything quickly goes from blurry and slow to sharp and crystalline.

And early indications suggest the team chose the right placebo. The last time I spoke to Polito, he was finding the majority of trial participants so far had assumed they were in the psilocybin group. Being a double-blinded trial, Polito and his team don't know who is getting the drug but, considering the cohort was half psilocybin/half placebo, it seemed to be a good sign the active placebo was working.

EVERY DAY? EVERY SECOND DAY?

Okay. We've sorted our dose and picked our active placebo. Now, what is the day-to-day protocol of microdosing?

Again, Polito came up against a truckload of discordant literature.[14] This, after all, has been an anecdotal phenomenon for a decade and people have been doing things in a wide variety of ways. Unsurprisingly, there is no *one right way* to microdose. And for every failed microdosing experiment, you can be sure to find an advocate of the practice simply argue that what was tested just wasn't the right way to do it.

The most popular protocol for microdosing was of course popularised by James Fadiman, the originator of the trend. He suggested the best way to go is to dose once every three days, for about a month, then take a break for a few weeks before starting the cycle again.

Mycologist Paul Stamets offers another popular microdosing strategy. Dubbed the 'Stamets Stack', he proposes a specific combination of psilocybin mushrooms, lion's mane mushroom and niacin. (Stamets has patented this special microdosing blend and is selling it – minus the psilocybin, of course – through his website. Psychedelic capitalism at its best.) You take this daily for four days, then take three days off, before repeating the loop for about a month. Again, his strategy recommends a break for a few weeks before resuming the protocol.

Generally, the world of microdosing is a motley mix of dissonant opinions. One survey asking more than 1000 microdosers how they took their doses found around 50 per cent simply made it up as they went along. The only relatively consistent thing to be found was most microdosers recommended taking regular breaks from dosing, usually every four to six weeks.[15] Microdosing isn't a thing you do all the time.

Polito ultimately settled on looking at the effects of psilocybin twice a week for six weeks. The twice-a-week part was an easy decision; this kind of strategy is easily the most common among microdosers. And, pragmatically, twice a week works well for a clinical trial context. Due to the still-illegal nature of psilocybin, patients would not be able to take the drugs home with them, so asking someone to come in twice a week is more reasonable than any kind of long-term daily offering.

Running each participant for six weeks, however, was perhaps a more complicated choice. 'I've been quite critical of short studies,' Polito told me emphatically. 'Because I don't think that they map onto the way that people really microdose.' In other words, there was no point going to this effort just to track someone dosing for two or three weeks.

Polito used conventional antidepressants as a useful comparator in focusing on six weeks; we know it is usually around the four-to-six-week point that clinicians have a good idea whether an antidepressant is going to be helpful to a patient. If this kind of microdosing protocol was going to be effective, then six weeks should be long enough to get some kind of signal. 'Having that longer time frame would just give us that extra certainty and extra chance to find an effect,' Polito explained. 'By week six, that's enough for you to be able to say, "Okay, there is something clinically meaningful happening here."'

It's also worth, at this point, acknowledging the elephant in the room: money. We'll get to the economics in a moment, but every extra day on the protocol adds exceptional amounts of cost to the trial as a whole. Six weeks, two doses a week, plus screening and miscellaneous visits means every single participant is coming to the trial site around 15 times over a two-month period. This adds up to big numbers. The clinical trial was not going to be cheap.

MICRODOSING FOR WHAT? CREATIVITY? MOOD? DEPRESSION?

As Polito's early field studies revealed, people microdose for a diverse array of reasons. And often those reasons don't necessarily match up with what users end up experiencing. What things should a microdosing trial be specifically testing for?

A crucial foundation in modern clinical trial research is the idea of the primary outcome. This is the single, directing hypothesis guiding most decisions behind the construction of a protocol. A trial can certainly incorporate an array of secondary outcomes, scales and measures, but the primary objective is crucial. Without a clear primary objective, researchers can often succumb to bias and cherry-picking. Maybe they saw no effect from their intervention on two or three different psychiatric scales, but there was one in particular that showed big results. Without a pre-selected primary measure, a researcher could ignore all the data they accrue showing nothing and just focus on the one thing that *did* show an effect.

A controversial example of this scenario took place in early 2021 when *The New England Journal of Medicine* published a study reporting on the results of a trial comparing the efficacy of psilocybin therapy for depression against common SSRI antidepressant treatment.[16] The trial's design was reasonably robust. Researchers recruited around 60 people with major depression and split them into two groups. One cohort received two big doses of psilocybin, three weeks apart, while taking a daily placebo and doing routine therapy sessions. The other group received placebo (1-milligram) psilocybin doses, while taking daily SSRI medication and also getting the routine therapy.

The primary outcome measure in the trial was a change in baseline scores on a widely used scale for measuring depression called the Quick Inventory of Depressive Symptomatology – Self-Report (QIDS-SR). At the end of the six-week trial, improvements were seen in both psilocybin and SSRI groups' QIDS-SR scores; however, no statistically significant differences were found. Basically, according to the QIDS-SR scores, psilocybin therapy was virtually as effective as the common antidepressant after six weeks of treatment.

Where this story starts to get a little unconventional is in the way the trial lead Robin Carhart-Harris went on a social media tirade in the weeks before the journal published the article.[17] Carhart-Harris delivered a 45-tweet-long spiel claiming the journal edited his article to present the results as conservative. He also claimed a figure showing how effective the psilocybin treatment was compared to the SSRI on ten different measures was pushed out of the main article and into the appendix against his wishes.

Looking at all the secondary data certainly painted a different picture of the trial, that's for sure. Several other depression and anxiety scales suggested psilocybin was way more effective than SSRI treatment, but the journal was sticking to its guns, claiming the registered primary outcome is what is important, and highlighting any secondary measures amounted to cherry-picking data. The journal wasn't alone in its monomaniacal focus on the single primary outcome.

Kevin McConway, an emeritus professor of applied statistics at the Open University, suggested what Carhart-Harris saw as a conservative framing of his results were actually established scientific conventions designed to prevent research data from being skewed.[18] He went on to describe Carhart-Harris as being 'misleading' by pointing to values in an appendix and claiming those were the results we should be paying attention to.

Most media reports at the time took the positive spin on the study and ran with it, highlighting how much better psilocybin performed for depression compared to standard SSRI therapy. But for me, the whole stoush highlighted just how thorny research can be, especially when you are dealing with psychedelics. If you want a treatment to work, then you can usually find some kind of measure or scale to show a positive outcome.

For his microdosing trial, Vince Polito didn't have much hesitation in setting up a primary outcome looking at the effects of the practice on mild and moderate depression.

'You've got to set up your trial for something. And I think that's the thing that has the most potential implications for the importance of microdosing. If it can help with depression, then that's really important. We need better treatments for depression. It's a plausible outcome because lots of people anecdotally report improvements with depression.'

The scale Polito is using to measure depression is called the GRID-Hamilton Rating Scale for Depression (GRID-HAMD).[19] It's probably one of the most commonly used depression measures in clinical studies, and will offer decent insights into whether microdosing confers antidepressant properties.

Setting this primary outcome was a strategic decision for Polito from a research perspective. The focus gave the trial greater import in the eyes of both academic and commercial partners. And yes, this means microdosing at these levels might be ultimately deployed as a pharmaceutical medicine.

Alongside this primary measure, Polito is still capturing a whole raft of other measurements over the course of the trial. With participants coming into the centre so often, he saw the opportunity to gather as much data as possible. Depression reduction may be the general goal, but if psilocybin microdosing does anything else, Polito was determined to find out.

> We've got a large battery [of tests] to give us chances to find out about other potential benefits. So we're looking at other measures of psychopathology, we're looking at cognition and creativity, we're looking at social variables, and variables around beliefs and attitudes. We've got blood-based biomarkers we're looking at. There's a neuroimaging sub-study where we also look at brain activity in a subset of participants.
>
> We're also collecting some pharmacokinetic data. So we'll be able to have more clear information about the impact of these kind of low doses. We're looking at impairment. We put people in the driving simulator and things like that, to be able to say something about the degree to which these low doses impact cognition in ways that are relevant for real-world tasks, if there is impairment.

It may seem like an everything-but-the-kitchen-sink approach, but Polito has spent years studying the phenomenon of microdosing. Advocates of the practice claim it does many things, so alongside the primary antidepressant outcome, the trial's extraordinary array of data gathering is close to as definitive as you can get in a single research project. If 4 milligrams of psilocybin, taken twice a week for six weeks, does anything detectable at all in human subjects, then Polito is going to catch it.

WHAT ABOUT THE WHO?

Perhaps the final big question in planning a big clinical trial is who you will be recruiting – and, more importantly, who you will be excluding. Inclusion criteria will always focus on a trial's primary outcome. Here it's the antidepressant effect of microdosing in depressed subjects.

In a distinct change of focus, Polito was more interested in his trial looking at participants without the conventional, serious, treatment-resistant kind of depression most psychedelic research concentrates on. Instead, his recruitment process involves screening with a psychiatrist for very moderate levels of depression.

Those interested in participating need to fit into a particular rating window using the GRID-HAMD scale. Maybe they had long-term, previously diagnosed, issues with depression, or maybe they had never been to a doctor for any kind of mental health screening. It didn't matter. The key was participants were not too severely depressed according to the scale, but just depressed enough. A goldilocks zone of mild-to-moderate depression – so to speak.

This highly specific zone has meant lots of applicants wanting to be in the trial simply haven't fit the bill. In fact, so far, Polito estimates about 50 per cent of applicants fail the screening process. For one reason or another, they just aren't quite there.

Other than that, setting up clear safety criteria was one of the other main factors for applicants to the trial. The usual conservative factors are here. No history of personal or familial mental health issues like schizophrenia or bipolar. No one currently on antidepressants is allowed. And no one with lots of personal experience with psychedelics. That last one helps screen out subjects with higher levels of positive sentiments towards psychedelics.

The number of participants Polito is aiming to enrol is another especially unique part of the trial. Over the last few years, there have been a few emerging clinical trials testing microdosing. But almost all these trials have been either short in duration (looking at a small handful of doses over a week or two) or small in scale (looking at cohorts of less than 100 people).

In late 2025, the results of a big LSD microdosing trial leaked out into the research world. Across the ditch, in New Zealand, Suresh Muthukumaraswamy and colleagues had completed their own landmark microdosing clinical trial. This trial was testing LSD instead of psilocybin. Suresh's trial tracked with a protocol similar to Polito's in many ways, focusing on a primary outcome of antidepressant effect, and using twice-weekly doses for a stretch of eight weeks.

The first publication to come out of the trial was its Phase 2a results.[20] This was data from the initial stage of the study, before a placebo group was included. Only around 20 subjects were included in the publication but the results were striking. Depression scores in the cohort had dropped by almost 60 per cent by the end of the trial, and they held there for six months.

You can imagine how microdosing evangelists jumped on this data. 'Look!' they exclaimed. 'Microdosing works! And it keeps working even after you stop.'

Missed by the advocates proclaiming such wonderful results was the fact that this was merely the first wave of open-label data from a larger trial – meaning there wasn't yet any comparison to a placebo control. The real meat and potatoes of the study were in its next stage.

This Phase 2b part of the trial used three different kinds of placebo: two active (Ritalin or caffeine) and one inactive. Plus, it incorporated a 'self-selected psychologically beneficial activity' to be completed on dose days as a way of enhancing mindfulness and amplifying any potential placebo effect.

About two weeks after the initial positive study was published, the CEO of the company funding the trial unexpectedly posted the top-line results of the larger Phase 2b work.[21] There had been a massive turnaround from the earlier published data. Turns out LSD microdosing for depression didn't work at all. Or, to be more accurate, it worked – but no more effectively than placebo.

The data reveal showed both LSD and placebo cohorts dropped about 30 per cent on depression scales by the end of the eight-week trial. The blinding tricks were effective, and everyone pretty much improved by spending eight weeks doing some beneficial psychological activities and becoming a little more mindful about their mood.

The big difference between this LSD trial and Polito's work is the scale. Despite a magnificently robust trial design, the LSD research only ultimately recruited 89 participants. Split evenly between placebo and LSD groups, that is a decent but small cohort to build conclusions from.

Polito is going bigger with his trial. And in the spirit of doing this thoroughly, he is shooting for 250 participants in total. Even split between placebo and microdose, this notably large cohort makes his trial well-powered to deliver data unlike any other clinical study in the world. If his data echoes the New Zealand data, you could start to make a good case for microdosing being little more than a powerful placebo.

7500 TAXI TRIPS

The reality of how resource-intensive a trial like this is dawns on you when you sit in the 'control room' while a regular day plays out. A part-time psychiatrist sits in a dose room with one participant, guiding them through the procedure of taking their first dose. Another participant waits in a second room.

We'll call him Aaron (not his real name). He is young and softly spoken, and has never participated in a clinical trial before this one. Aaron first learned about psychedelics from a podcast. He started reading some of the science, dug around on Reddit, and became fascinated with the potential of these strange drugs. Searching for a clinical trial he could participate in to try them out, he stumbled across the Macquarie microdosing study.

After a longwinded screening process, he was finally enrolled, and when I met him he was on his third dosing day. Aaron is confident he's not in the placebo group. He tells me that within 25 minutes of his first dose, he felt a strange wave of happiness and joy. Lights became a little hazy but other than that he couldn't really discern any effects from the dose he would describe as 'psychedelic'. Any acute feelings from the microdose generally disappear by the next day but Aaron is excited to see if the process leads to any cumulative persistent benefits over the six-week cycle.

Being a blinded study, no one knows whether Aaron is right in his guess that he's in the psilocybin group. Maybe he's getting the placebo, and the transient benefits he senses are simply a caffeine buzz. If he is getting the placebo, then Polito's blinding strategy certainly is working.

After briefly chatting with Aaron, I return to the control room. Andy, the trial manager, is booking a taxi to pick Aaron up after his dose. Every participant gets two doses a week, dubbed A-dose and B-dose. The A-dose comprises a super short visit to the site, mainly to be given the pill and checked by the psychiatrist that everything is going fine. When participants get their B-dose, the researchers put them through some kind of test. Six weeks, six different tests. One week it could be having a go in a driving simulator, the next could be broad set of blood tests, and another could take the participant through a MEG scanner.

This was an A-dose for Aaron. So just a quick visit; in and out.

SPENDING TIME AT THE TRIAL SITE, I STARTED TO wonder: who was paying for all of this? Everywhere I looked, the dollars were adding up.

Taxi services, for example, are provided for every participant to and from the university hospital for every visit. All up, that's 250 subjects times 15 visits per subject. We have 3750 individual participant site visits, with two taxi trips for each visit. That's 7500 funded taxi trips the trial needs to account for. I hear the cash register chime a couple of hundred thousand dollars right there.

Then you have a psychiatrist working at least two full-time days a week, solely for the trial, for the better part of two or three years. A trial manager runs the admin side of things. A site space costs money, as do the drugs, storage and so on. All the bloodwork goes to labs and they charge for the results. Everything costs money. And all this just to gather hundreds of thousands of pages of raw data that will then need to be crunched and turned into interpretable results.

The trial itself, all up, will cost *millions* of dollars. Polito is reticent to give me an actual number but he nods at the 'millions' estimate, simply saying a study like this is 'ridiculously expensive'. And any quick calculation of the above will get you to some mind-boggling numbers.

This all takes time and money. Who pays for this?

When Polito was first sketching out his ideas for the trial, during the Covid years, it was a much smaller proposition. No one immediately shot for designing something on such a wildly expansive scale. But the psychedelic boom years in the early 2020s led to some big opportunities, and a burgeoning pharmaceutical company became interested in what Polito was doing.

This company was working on a proprietary formulation of psilocybin, initially developing a 1-milligram rapid-release capsule. The opportunity for both parties was huge. In Polito, the company saw a researcher perfectly placed to test their new drug – a drug which, if successful, could return untold amounts of money in the mental health pharma space. For Polito, he saw a company willing to fund not his small, narrow idea but the big moonshot: a large-scale clinical trial robust enough to fully test the potential of psilocybin microdosing.

Dealing with pharmaceutical companies and big money was a new experience for Polito, whose previous research had been small-scale cognitive science studies. The alternative was still there: a smaller study, maybe with some government funding. But in the case of microdosing, there were plenty of others doing those smaller investigations. Getting a cohort of 50 or even 100 people, giving them a handful of doses and doing a few tests along the way: what would that prove?

Here, Polito felt like he had a unique chance to do something relatively close to definitive, or as definitive as a single-site trial can ever be. Ultimately, his study is still what is known as an investigator-initiated trial, something he's proud to stress. This means that despite any external commercial funding, the development of the protocol is all his own, untouched by commercial demands, and the university is a primary sponsor. In the end, the results will be the results. A company may be stumping up the cash in the gamble that something positive is returned. But if it's a miss, then so be it.

'If we get to the end of this and we find null effects, I'll be pretty confident that, actually, microdosing doesn't help with depression,' Polito tells me. 'And if we find effects, then I think it would be pretty hard to ignore the findings from this study. So I'm really pleased with what we've set up and think either way the results are going to be important.'

I last visited the trial site in August 2025. The team was about 18 months into the work and estimated that it would be two more years before it would conclude. Maybe sometime in 2027 you'll see some data revealed. Maybe you'll see a news headline in early 2028 suggesting psilocybin microdosing does or doesn't work. You'll spend 60 seconds scanning the article, noting the results, then move onto the next thing.

But know that brief moment of your time took Vince Polito five years and millions of dollars to conclude. Clinical research is hard. Psychedelic studies are even harder.

4

DMT

LONG TRIPS. SHORT TRIPS. NO TRIPS.

'I don't take drugs. I am the drug.'

Salvador Dalí, quoted in Javier Pérez Andújar,
Salvador Dalí: A la conquista de lo irracional, Algaba, 2003

'It started when I was travelling through South America, meeting people that had taken ayahuasca who were reporting these incredible benefits. Decades on antidepressants with severe depression, and then after three ceremonies they're throwing their medications in the river and feeling incredible.'

Daniel Perkins had already traversed a diverse academic career in the mental health space before bumping up against the psychedelic world in 2015. His PhD project at the turn of the millennium looked at how social interventions could help long-term unemployed people with severe mental health problems. Back then, Perkins was struck with just how difficult it was to bring about change in a person battling psychiatric challenges.

He subsequently worked with the Victorian government on broader mental health strategy, and was at the forefront of the country's medical cannabis work, both in regulation and research.

All these interests coalesced during a trip around Peru. It was his introduction to ayahuasca. The massive transformative change people were experiencing from this psychedelic brew was strikingly unusual and initially Perkins was a little sceptical. Were these people really getting lasting improvements to their mental health, or were they just going back to their home countries and then crashing into a psychological crisis? Surely the extreme benefits he was seeing would be short-lived.

When Perkins got back to Australia, he started pulling together a team with similar interests at the University of Melbourne. Alongside colleague Jerome Sarris, Perkins was eager to understand whether his anecdotal observations from Peru were real.

Their first work was epidemiological. The team collected as much data as they could on who was using ayahuasca, what benefits they were seeing, and what types of broader psychological outcomes were emerging in the days, weeks and months after taking the traditional brew.

'The data we were collecting was sort of substantiating the claims that I was hearing back in Peru of these very dramatic life-transformative therapeutic benefits being reported by people – and it seemed to be pretty sustained. It also was occurring in the context of this broader enhancement of wellbeing, of self-perception and self-efficacy.'

By 2020, Perkins and his colleagues were convinced they were on to something that could help a lot of people with mental health issues. Here was a treatment that really generated those transformative changes clinicians had sought in mental health therapy. But how could such a unique concoction like ayahuasca become a medicine used by doctors in Western clinics? And what was in ayahuasca anyway?

ANTHROPOLOGISTS AND BOTANISTS HAVE KNOWN about ayahuasca (pronounced *eye-ah-waska*) for hundreds of years. Jesuit missionaries were some of the earliest Westerners to chronicle the traditional ceremony, describing indigenous users disparagingly as 'liars and sorcerers'.[1] In the early 1850s a famous British botanist named Richard Spruce was first to scientifically catalogue the psychoactive potion.

Spending years traversing vast stretches of the Amazon, Spruce frequently came across indigenous people engaging with this ceremonial brew. He noted the ayahuasca was always consumed in a ritualistic context with a divinatory framework. As a psychedelic experience, ayahuasca is long – lasting six to eight hours – and often involves periods of distinctive physical discomfort. Spruce noted one ingredient common across most preparations: a particular woody vine he named *Banisteria caapi* (later renamed *Banisteriopsis caapi*).

For the next hundred years, ayahuasca remained a pharmacological mystery. The caapi vine was thoroughly analysed but chemists struggled to understand what compounds were responsible for the brew's hallucinogenic effects.

Two key alkaloids were identified in the vine: harmine and harmaline. But when bold researchers tested the drugs on themselves, they struggled to get any kind of powerful psychoactive experience. Sure, the molecules were mildly mind-altering, but they were nothing like what was being reported and witnessed in the Amazon jungles when real ayahuasca was imbibed. What else was in the mix?

The popular scientific origin story for ayahuasca is that the mysterious secret ingredient wasn't discovered until the mid-1960s, when a student ethnobotanist named Homer Pinkley was embedded in a small village in Ecuador.[2] The morning after a local ceremony, Pinkley dug around in the cauldron used to prepare the potion the night before. Finding a few unidentified leaves, Pinkley took the samples and discovered they were from a plant called *Psychotria viridis*, a shrub commonly found in the Amazon that carries high concentrations of a psychedelic drug known as DMT (*N,N*-dimethyltryptamine).

The story of DMT gives us a compelling frame to understand how psychedelics can possibly become modern psychiatric medicines. As we'll see, depending on how it is consumed, DMT can lead to either extraordinarily long psychedelic journeys or profoundly short out-of-body experiences. This has made it the perfect substance to serve as a testing ground for questions around how long a psychedelic experience needs to last to be therapeutically effective.

But let's start at the beginning of Western science's strange journey with DMT. Despite popular accounts, Homer Pinkley wasn't the first person to shine a light on this DMT-containing Amazonian plant. That honour goes to none other than infamous beat generation writer William S Burroughs, who 15 years prior had gone on his own personal journey into the Amazon in search of what he dubbed the 'final fix'.

THE FINAL FIX

In 1951, William Burroughs was living in Mexico City, technically on the run from a drug possession charge in the United States.[3] It was here he shot his wife, Joan Vollmer, in the head.

Two years into the couple's Mexico jaunt, their days were spent in drug and alcohol stupors. One evening, at a friend's apartment among a rowdy collection of drunks, Burroughs suggested he and his wife play an impromptu William Tell game. Except instead of an apple and a crossbow, Burroughs pulled out a cheap handgun and urged his wife to put a glass on her head.

Moments later, Vollmer was on the floor in a pool of blood and Burroughs ended up in a Mexican jail charged with manslaughter. For the next 18 months, a distraught Burroughs suffered an existential crisis. He remembered reading about a mysterious 'lurid narcotic' called yagé, the world's most powerful psychoactive drug.[4] So he set out in search of this mystery hallucinogen, hoping to find a drug that could purge him of the 'ugly spirit' he associated with the killing of his wife.

This mission would ultimately turn into an eight-month gonzo anthropological journey through South America, chronicled in his and Allen Ginsberg's semi-fictional book *The Yage Letters,* published nearly 15 years later.

Fortuitously, within days of his arrival in Bogotá at the beginning of his venture, Burroughs met an equally mad mind in ethnobotanist Richard Evan Schultes. Since 1941, Schultes had been working among the native peoples of Colombia, cataloguing thousands of novel plants and finding at least half a dozen psychoactive compounds entirely new to Western science. Schultes, of course, had also tried all these drugs personally. So he and Burroughs got along just fine.

Initially guided by Schultes, Burroughs travelled from Colombia to Peru and back looking for a true yagé experience. Several underwhelming psychedelic experiences led him to question the yagé recipe. He spent weeks concocting his own psychoactive brews from a personal stash of caapi vine before definitively concluding something else must be in the mix – something that was being kept secret.

Eventually, Burroughs ended up in a small eastern Peruvian town called Pucallpa. He was introduced to a young local medicine man who was happy to offer Burroughs yagé. And this time Burroughs quickly realised he had finally been given a dose of the real thing. In a letter to friend Allen Ginsberg, he enthusiastically called yagé the most powerful drug he had ever experienced.

'Hold the presses! Everything I wrote about Yage subject to revision in the light of subsequent experience. It is not like weed, nor anything else I have ever experienced. I am now prepared to believe the Brujos [a term often used to represent a darker side to the local shaman or healer] do have secrets, and that Yage alone is quite different from Yage prepared with the leaves and plants the Brujos add to it.'[5]

After a couple more ceremonial experiences, Burroughs was finally shown how it was made. A second leafy plant was added to the caapi vine during the boiling. Burroughs picked a few leaves from this mystery plant before heading back to his home base in Florida.

In December 1954 Burroughs sent Schultes a Christmas card with notes on his discovery. The card also contained samples of the mystery plant Burroughs was certain would unlock the mystery of ayahuasca.[6] Schultes never replied to Burroughs' letters, simply storing the plant in his archives, unexamined.

By 1967, Homer Pinkley, one of Schultes' student anthropologists, had finally revealed the mystery of ayahuasca. *Psychotria viridis* was the secret ingredient, Schultes proudly declared at an ethnopharmacology meeting in San Francisco. A couple of years later, as a footnote in an article about the origins of ayahuasca, Schultes mentioned in passing that an earlier sample of *P. viridis* had been potentially gathered by Burroughs, but it wasn't until 1973 that anyone actually grabbed the old leaves out of a box for proper identification. And even then, the full story of Burroughs' involvement wasn't uncovered until 2017, when academic Andrew Lees dug up some previously unpublished letters between Burroughs and Schultes.[7]

We now understand that the pharmacological magic of ayahuasca involves a unique interplay between DMT in the *P. viridis* leaves and harmala molecules in the *Banisteriopsis caapi* vine. You see, if you eat or drink anything containing DMT by itself, you will feel nothing. An enzyme in your gut called monoamine oxidase quickly puts a stop to DMT getting into your bloodstream and then your brain. But harmala molecules block the activity of this enzyme, so when you mix something containing harmala with something containing DMT, you suddenly create a potent drinkable brew that leads to hours and hours of psychedelic visions.

And, as we'll soon learn, the duration of a psychedelic trip may be key to the drug's therapeutic benefits. A long trip may be important.

THE CRITICAL PERIOD

In mid-2023 an extraordinary study was published in the prestigious journal *Nature*.[8] The researchers were trying to understand how psychedelics exert their beneficial therapeutic effects. Psychedelics are being investigated for a wide variety of mental health issues (from anxiety and depression to post-traumatic stress disorder and addiction), but *how* do they help such a disparate array of problems?

Looking for some kind of common neurological mechanism, the work centred around an idea known as 'the critical period'. For decades scientists have recognised that when we are very young, our brains have a remarkable malleability. In the first few years of life especially, our brains are developing wildly fast. Synaptic connections are constantly forming, re-forming and shifting in a way that is often described as 'neuroplasticity'.

As we get older we lose this youthful plasticity and our neural circuits become more fixed. And some have hypothesised that a key underlying factor in many mental health problems could be an excess of fixed dysfunctional neural circuits. For a long time, neuroscientists have sought to develop drugs that can restore neuroplasticity to the brain to help treat psychiatric disorders.

The 2023 research, led by a team from Johns Hopkins University, wondered if one of the universal beneficial therapeutic mechanisms of psychedelics was they can temporarily reopen these critical periods of brain plasticity. Prior study from the same team found it likely that this was one of the key therapeutic mechanisms underpinning the efficacy of MDMA therapy for post-traumatic stress disorder. But what about psychedelics?

The big headline finding was that psychedelics do indeed seem to reopen this critical period. The researchers tested a variety of different psychedelic drugs that have recently been explored for therapeutic uses: psilocybin, LSD, ketamine and ibogaine. And, across a series of mouse experiments, they found all four drugs triggered similar youthful behaviours that are known to correlate with critical-period plasticity.

But even more curious was the finding that different drugs seemed to reopen those critical periods for different durations.

The foundational knowledge we have, from several prior studies, is looking at ketamine. We know ketamine has an effective and fast antidepressant effect, but the therapeutic benefits don't last very long – a week or two at best.

Ketamine's subjective effects (aka 'the trip') last anywhere from 30 to 90 minutes. And the Johns Hopkins team discovered that ketamine reopens the brain's critical period for about 48 hours. So a trip that lasts about an hour keeps a critical period of neuroplasticity open for a couple of days.

Looking at the other drugs on the same measures was where things got super interesting. The duration of a drug's subjective effect perfectly correlated with the duration each drug opened the mouse brain's critical period. The longer the 'trip', the longer the brain's critical period remained open.

Psilocybin, with a three-to-six-hour trip, kept the mouse brain in a critical period state for around two weeks. LSD, a slightly longer trip than psilocybin, led to an open critical period of three weeks, and ibogaine (an infamously long psychedelic that can generate a trip lasting anywhere from 12 to 36 hours) opened the critical period for over four weeks.

And these measures then correlated with the durability of each drug's therapeutic effect. In simple terms, the study was suggesting the length of a subjective drug trip could be directly related to how long one may feel therapeutic benefits. An hour or two and you may be better for a few weeks, but a longer trip from, say, LSD or ibogaine, and those improvements could hold strong for months, or even years. And this all comes down to the strange association between a trip's duration and the time a critical period of neuroplasticity remains open in the weeks following.

PHARMA-HUASCA

In 2021 entrepreneurial investors around the world were throwing money at any and every psychedelic project being floated. Daniel Perkins describes it as a 'psychedelic bubble'. Emails were coming to Perkins, from out of the blue, with offers of big money. Everyone wanted to get involved in his work. By the middle of the year, his team had launched the Psychae Institute in Melbourne, a not-for-profit research centre looking to develop pharmaceutical therapies based on the unique properties of a DMT–harmala combination. The treatment was informally nicknamed pharma-huasca, or ayahuasca in a pill.

So why did Perkins think a DMT–harmala combination therapy could be useful when there was already plenty of research into other similar longer-acting psychedelics like psilocybin and LSD?

Well, first there seemed to be a relatively unique duration to DMT–harmala combinations. Psilocybin generally results in an experience of four to six hours; LSD can be slightly longer than that. But Perkins' novel formulation sat more in the three-to-five-hour window of psychoactive effects. In theory, that timeframe was a little easier to work with in terms of modern nine-to-five medical clinics.

More than that, though, Perkins had an intriguing hypothesis. What if all classic psychedelics were not interchangeable? What if psilocybin, LSD and DMT all did different things to the brain? And what if the different qualities of psychedelic experiences generated by each of these drugs led to different therapeutic outcomes? Basically, what if a pharma-huasca combination was more therapeutically effective than other classic psychedelics?

His team's anthropological data seemed to suggest this might be the case. Those transformative life changes Perkins knew were crucial to patients gaining lasting improvements seemed to be more reliably generated by ayahuasca compared to psilocybin or LSD. He noticed the extended DMT experience, potentiated by the harmala combination, offered patients a type of autobiographical trip that turned out to be especially useful in triggering big life changes.

'With the DMT–harmala combination, people – say, with addictions – often have this deep understanding of what was the real root cause of their addiction, [and] how that has cascaded through different things over their lives, how it might have affected other people,' Perkins explains to me. 'And then also this change in self-deception and desire to actually look after their own health. A lot of that comes from this psychedelic experience, and the insights they're getting and the new understandings.'

So the first step in Perkins' research journey was finding out what kind of combination of harmala and DMT worked best to get patients into deep psychedelic states. That study, conducted at Melbourne's St Vincent's Hospital across early 2023, recruited nine people, all with prior ayahuasca experience.[9]

Two mixes were first tested, based on DMT extracts derived from different Australian acacia sources – as we'll soon discover, DMT can be found in an extraordinary array of plants, including some iconic native Australian flora. Initial subjective ratings from participants suggested the psychedelic effects were a little weak compared to their prior ayahuasca experiences, so a third mix was developed. And the team upped the concentrations. Mystical experience ratings skyrocketed for the small cohort who were given high doses of this third mix. All regarded this combination as equal to, or in some cases stronger, than any traditional ayahuasca experience they'd had.

Perkins and his team had found their pharma-huasca mix.

Looking forward, the team are now moving onto what is known as a PK/PD (pharmacokinetic/pharmacodynamic) study. This is a first-phase human trial that robustly tracks what a drug is doing inside a human body. Before completing any larger human trial testing a drug's clinical use, scientists need to know how that drug is metabolised by a body and what people experience when taking the drug.

If all goes to plan, Perkins and colleagues will have that data promptly, leading to more thorough clinical trials testing their unique ayahuasca pill in patients by the end of 2027.

And Perkins is far from the only researcher exploring the ways DMT can be used in modern medicine. You see, DMT is a really unusual drug. In ayahuasca it generates a long, deep, multi-hour experience, but that's not the only way it can be consumed. When smoked, or snorted or injected, it does something completely different – something quick, weird, and thoroughly unlike any other classic psychedelic. I know, because when I was younger I tried it.

ZEN IN A CRACK PIPE

In my twenties I thought of myself as a defiant counterculture operative. I pushed up against 'consensus reality' with a kind of youthful know-it-all vigour that only really exists when you are old enough to be independent but still too young to understand how the world works. I was against anything 'mainstream', and fought against the mind virus of popular culture. I was putting on parties as part of the Aussie 'doof' scene and doing the whole DJ thing whenever I got the chance. It was a whole scene, man.

All this ultimately led me to a point where one day I was sitting by a stream in a lush rainforest about to smoke DMT for the very first time. I'd read my share of psychedelic literature and thought I was prepared for what was to come. Or as prepared as you can be for something as ineffable as DMT. What was unexpected, in the moment, was an odd discordance between the beauty of the surrounding nature and the strange modern paraphernalia needed to imbibe the drug.

Bright-orange crystals of pure DMT were carefully dropped into the head of a glass pipe, the type of pipe my brain only really associated with movies about urban crack smoking. A jet lighter blasted the pipe. Inhale deeply, I was instructed. Hold it, and now inhale again. The smoke tasted acrid. I coughed.

Needless to say, the experience was memorable, but not in the way you might think. I don't remember a great deal about the moments immediately after inhaling the drug. And if I did, I'd spare you from reading a handful of paragraphs where an author uses their most flowery prose to describe the indescribable. No, we're not going to talk about fractals or interdimensional travel.

What has stuck with me over the nearly 20 years since this experience are the ways the days *felt* after that incredibly short time in the forest. The DMT experience couldn't have lasted more than 20 minutes, but the ripple inside me lingered for weeks.

I was never a particularly anxious or irritable person, at least in my twenties. Nevertheless, even at those more emotionally settled points in my life, I was always a bit of a contrary curmudgeon. Little things frustrated me. I was the annoying guy at a party keen to poke holes in whatever world view was being espoused. Studying postmodern philosophy in my undergrad years probably didn't help. I was a little like a real-life internet troll, except before that was a really awful thing.

For a few weeks after that DMT experience, I felt a kind of internal calm that was profoundly unusual. I remember jokingly calling the drug 'Zen in a crack pipe'. Nothing bothered me. Everything was fine. Deadlines weren't a stress. 'We'll figure it out,' I said. 'Don't worry about it,' I'd hear myself say.

It was such a distinct feeling that I remember it to this very day. It didn't last forever. At some point the 'Larry David' in me slowly returned, but I never forgot the sense that this drug had done something to my brain that was sublime.

What happened in my brain that day? Were the strangely calming effects I felt over the following weeks simply the result of some kind of pharmacological mechanism? Did the drug temporarily flick a switch in some brain receptors causing a weeks-long anti-anxiety sensation? Or was there something more philosophically ground-shaking going on?

IT'S EVERYWHERE AND IN EVERYTHING

DMT, or *N,N*-dimethyltryptamine, is by far the weirdo child in our diverse family of classic psychedelics. The other kids have relatively straightforward backgrounds. Psilocybin comes from a particular group of mushrooms. Mescaline is rarer, found in just a handful of cacti species. And LSD is even more specific, a unique, semi-synthetic molecule tweaked from a natural substance found in a type of ergot fungus known to infect grain.

DMT, on the other hand, can be found everywhere in nature. The molecule has been detected in flowers, trees, grasses and even animals. In fact, once scientists started looking for it, they even found DMT inside the human body. It is the only psychedelic substance naturally produced within us.

And we don't know why it's there or what it is doing.

The chemical was first synthesised back in the early 1930s by a Canadian chemist who was playing around with different tryptamines. At that point it was just noted as a molecular curiosity but never tested for anything. A few years later a Brazilian microbiologist found DMT in the bark of a common tree fern. The plant was used by local indigenous people in a variety of ways but at the time the molecule was never suspected to be especially psychoactive.

By the early 1950s, as we know, scientists had started looking everywhere for new psychedelic drugs. A trio of American chemists explicitly homed in on DMT while analysing compounds from a traditional psychoactive snuff in the Amazon. But still, at this point, no human had directly experimented with pure DMT.

Over in Hungary, a physician named Stephen Szára was trying to get an order of LSD from the labs of Sandoz in Switzerland.[10] The world was in the thick of the Cold War, and Sandoz politely refused his request. The company was not comfortable sending such an experimental psychoactive drug across the Iron Curtain. So Szára began digging around chemistry journals to see what else he could find. He was fascinated by the emerging studies linking DMT with traditional South American rituals, so he put his chemistry skills to the test and swiftly synthesised 10 grams of the drug.

Using himself as a guinea pig, Szára started taking oral doses of DMT to see if the chemical was actually psychedelic. Starting low, and taking larger doses everyday, Szára quickly got up to massive volumes of nearly a gram at a time without feeling any effects. Maybe this wasn't the psychedelic culprit he was looking for? Just as he was about to move on and try something else, a colleague suggested he inject the drug to see what happens.

So, in April 1956, Szára tested a tiny dose of pure DMT injected into his muscle. He quickly felt something: geometric swirls appeared when he closed his eyes. A couple of days later, he tried again with a bigger dose.

Bang! Within minutes he was transported somewhere else, and that was DMT's introduction to the Western world.

Knowledge of Szára's experiences quickly filtered down through the grapevine of research chemists and psychonauts, but for the next few decades DMT remained a resolutely niche psychedelic. It didn't have the general appeal of its cousins LSD or psilocybin. For one, you needed to smoke or inject it to get any effects. And, perhaps most significantly, it had nearly no recreational value. It came on fast, within seconds sometimes, took its user to a different reality altogether for half an hour, and then returned them back to Earth. This wasn't a party drug. Or even a revolutionary counterculture drug. It was something else.

IN THE 21ST CENTURY RENAISSANCE OF PSYCHEDELIC science, it seemed inevitable that researchers would eventually begin to explore DMT as a medicine. Despite the recent 'critical period' findings, the idea of a shorter trip makes for a more scalable modern medical treatment. After all, if doctors can turn dosing days into a swift 90-minute clinic visit, then psychedelic medicine becomes a lot less resource-intensive. Why trip for hours when you could get similar benefits from something quicker? Maybe you need to take it more often, but that doesn't matter. In the 21st century, many people will sacrifice a bit of efficacy for something easier, faster. This could be a drug you take on your lunch break.

Nasal-spray formulations of DMT are certainly in the works. Daniel Perkins and his team are already working on something like this alongside their longer-acting harmala combination. His hypothesis is that not all psychiatric conditions may need a long, introspective trip. For some mental health conditions – maybe anxiety or mild depression – a shorter-acting psychedelic could be just as effective.[11] A little mental shake-up could be all you need.

Except with DMT there is one unusual problem. A problem that complicates turning this into a widely used mainstream medicine.

That problem … is interdimensional elves …

THE MACHINE ELVES

'I was neither intellectually nor emotionally prepared for the frequency with which contact with beings occurred in our studies, nor the often utterly bizarre nature of these experiences,' wrote psychiatrist Rick Strassman, whose five-year experiment with DMT in the early 1990s pushed the boundaries of what a scientific study can do. 'Neither, it seemed, were many of the volunteers, even those who had smoked DMT previously. Also surprising were the common themes of what these beings were doing with so many of our volunteers: manipulating, communicating, showing, helping, questioning. It was definitely a two-way street.'[12]

Strassman is the true, unheralded pioneer of the modern psychedelic renaissance. Between December 1988 and November 1990, he traversed a Kafkaesque bureaucracy to get approval for a unique experiment. He wanted to rigorously chronicle exactly what happened when healthy human beings were injected with DMT.

The oft-told story of the psychedelic renaissance in the early 2000s tends to focus on Roland Griffiths, a psychopharmacologist at the Johns Hopkins School of Medicine in Baltimore, whose experiments with psilocybin are generally seen as the beginning of the modern renaissance of psychedelic research. But Griffiths was not the first researcher in our modern era to get governmental approval to work with psychedelic drugs. The first was Strassman, whose work with DMT preceded Griffiths' research by more than a decade.

Strassman's proposal was deceptively simple. His work on the pineal gland – a tiny, hormone-secreting gland in the centre of the brain – had led him to a wild hypothesis: that near-death and mystical experiences are both linked to a release of DMT from this gland. The first step in studying this hypothesis would be to administer DMT to a cohort of healthy participants and see if their experiences in any way resembled what others had recorded in near-death research. Anecdotally, people who had gone through near-death experiences tended to recount stories that Strassman felt were similar to how DMT is talked about: white lights, travelling to another place, feelings of calm, meeting other beings.

After two years of miraculous regulatory wrangling, Strassman became the first person in 20 years to legally give someone psychedelic drugs in the United States. For the next five years, he worked with 60 volunteers, administering around 400 doses of DMT. The work ended in 1995 and Strassman published a handful of studies along the way, reporting on minor things like technical dose-response data.

It wasn't until 2001, with the publication of his book *DMT: The Spirit Molecule*, that the true extent of the weirdness around Strassman's research was revealed. The book extensively detailed the experiences of his volunteers during the five-year study, and it's fair to say his sense of scientific objectivity was thoroughly challenged by the end of the experiment.

As the experiment progressed, Strassman began noticing participants in the study were reporting oddly similar experiences. These weren't the abstract kaleidoscopic visions many talk about when taking psychedelic drugs like psilocybin or LSD. They also weren't memory-laced flashbacks or autobiographical visions of their childhood. Instead, people were telling Strassman the drug was transporting them to a tangible space, an 'alien realm' as real as the world we inhabit. And once there, they were making contact with a distinct kind of intelligent being. Terms like 'elves', 'insects' and 'aliens' were often used by participants as they tried to describe these entities.

Many participants in the study had prior experience with psychedelics. They were well attuned to the difference between hallucination and reality. However, these experienced psychonauts all were clear in describing their DMT journeys as notably 'unpsychedelic' and highly detailed. 'We all dream of unusual places and things,' Strassman wrote in his iconic book:

> However, our volunteers not only saw these things, but felt an unshakeable certainty that they actually were there. Opening their eyes at any time superimposed this reality with their now-manifest but previously invisible one. Neither were they asleep. They were hyperaware and awake, able to tell themselves to do things in this new space. It's amazing how often I heard them say, 'I looked around and saw ...'[13]

Perhaps more extraordinary was that Strassman's reports were not novel. Connections between elvish or insectoid entities and DMT go back to the very first reported experiences with the drug. Stephen Szára wrote about similar encounters with interdimensional beings when he was first giving human volunteers DMT injections in the 1950s. Timothy Leary called the entities 'magnificent insects' when he was finally given the drug, while renowned psychonaut Terence McKenna famously wrote about his encounters with 'machine elves'. Even William Burroughs called the entities 'Soulless Insect People' after getting his hands on pure DMT in the early 1960s.

Strassman ultimately abandoned his research in 1995. Alongside funding and personnel issues, he began to have some ethical concerns about the work. He was rarely seeing participants gain any long-term benefits from the DMT sessions, perhaps due to the lack of any associated psychological care. And some people's experiences were proving hard to integrate into their normal lives. The places they had travelled to seemed so real. What if they *had* actually gone somewhere else?

'Listening to these experiences also began stretching my limits as a clinical psychiatrist and researcher,' Strassman admitted:

> I made few comments regarding people's reports of these unseen realms. It was hard to keep up, and I didn't know what to say. It was at this point that I began having to fight a tendency to regard these stories as dreams, or figments of their DMT-amplified imaginations. On the other hand, I also began doubting my own model for what exactly happens on DMT. Were people really somewhere else? What exactly were they witnessing?[14]

Strassman's findings were likely too weird for mainstream science to process. The work slipped into the footnotes of psychedelic history. Even Strassman himself spent the rest of his career trying to grapple with what he saw in those DMT years. His work presented a massive ontological dilemma to modern psychedelic scientists.

Even if DMT did seem to have some kind of beneficial therapeutic effect, how could this inconvenient side effect of interdimensional travel be managed? And what could medical professionals say to patients when they gave them a medicine that reliably triggers an encounter with non-human entities?

This may seem like a fringe question, but it is one modern researchers have struggled with. A 2015 study encompassing 800 psychedelic users found more than one in three people had experienced 'encounters with spiritual entities' after taking DMT.[15] An even more thorough investigation by a team from Johns Hopkins, published in 2020, surveyed more than 2500 people who had come across entities after imbibing DMT. This incredible study characterised a number of different types of entity encounters; it found that 69 per cent of experiences included the participant being given some kind of personal message to take back to their normal life. The vast majority of reports described the encounter as 'more real than everyday waking consciousness' and fewer than 25 per cent of respondents suggested the entity was merely a figment of their imagination.[16]

Okay, so the entities are just good guys wanting to help out, and everyone coming back from a DMT trip reports positive experiences, right?

Not exactly. Of those people reporting entity contact with DMT, around one in ten returned with deeply negative experiences. This group called the entities 'malevolent'. Another ayahuasca survey found 15 per cent of users reported feeling 'energetically attacked' after a psychedelic experience.[17]

Psychedelic harm minimisation researcher Jules Evans suggests this is a problem that many modern psychedelic medical advocates are trying to sweep under the rug. From Evans' perspective, it is hard to argue malevolent entities aren't an issue with psychedelic medicine; after all, the empirical data is clear. A significant proportion of people who take psychedelics (particularly DMT and ayahuasca) encounter entities, and if we accept this to be something people should be warned about, then Evans argues that

> it becomes difficult to see psychedelic medicine ever moving from the New Age subculture to mainstream healthcare without a revolution in the Western world view.
>
> It's hard to imagine the FDA including 'risk of spirit possession' in its labelling. And I think it would be off-putting to many potential ordinary-Joe consumers if you told them, 'Take this pill and there's a good chance you might encounter benevolent entities, but perhaps a one-in-ten chance they could be malevolent.' Who'd want to go in the ocean if 10 per cent of the fish attacked you?

What if there was a way to avoid this whole entity problem altogether? What if there was a short-acting psychedelic similar to DMT that didn't send users into another dimension to talk to aliens, but instead just dissolved the entire world into nothing? Maybe *that* could be more useful as our lunchtime depression medicine?

THE FIRST AUSTRALIAN CLINICAL PSYCHEDELIC RESEARCH LAB

Like many players in Australia's psychedelic renaissance, Paul Liknaitzky spent years circling the idea of working with hallucinogenic drugs but he always had to approach the topic indirectly. Starting his academic path in neuroscience before crossing the Rubicon into psychology with his PhD, Liknaitzky was consistently and fundamentally interested in the idea of altered states of consciousness.

More specifically, his curiosity led him to look at what kinds of commonalities were shared by a variety of different induction techniques into what some researchers have dubbed 'non-ordinary states of consciousness', or NSCs. Of course, psychedelics can trigger an NSC, but so can an assortment of other non-drug experiences, from the 'high' long-distance runners often talk about, to the deep state of mindfulness reached in serious meditation practice.

Not only was Liknaitzky interested in the neuroscience of these practices but his focus quickly ended up investigating their clinical utility. How do these NSCs work to benefit those suffering from clinical depression? What is it about depression that seems to respond to certain kinds of altered states of consciousness but not others?

His thesis ultimately presented a new kind of overarching

explanation for depression dubbed the Hyper-ordinary Depression Hypothesis. Here Liknaitzky suggested many accounts of depression are characterised by a kind of rigidity in thinking that one is unable to escape. In contrast, the triggering of an NSC can alleviate some symptoms of depression, be it through acts of physical endurance, meditation or psychedelic drugs.

For Liknaitzky, the idea was a culmination of a lifetime's thinking about suffering, existence and all the big ideas. From a young age he had personally experienced how meditation could dramatically alter his own mental state. As a clinician, the lure of psychedelics being able to quickly trigger those meaningful experiences in patients was like catnip. But the idea of actually working with psychedelics in a serious academic context was still wildly fringe.

He finished his PhD at the end of 2016 and for the next few years bided his time, but by late 2019 he was sensing a wave building. Some colleagues at Monash University in Melbourne were keen to jump into the world of psychedelic research and he was more than ready. The will was there, but where was the money?

The web of connections ended up leading Liknaitzky to a meeting with an Australian cannabis company. They were keen to get some skin in the psychedelic game, so to speak. Liknaitzky was poised to make his pitch: a trial testing psilocybin for generalised anxiety. The company was keen, Liknaitzky had the protocol, and the university was on board.

It was 2020 and things were moving fast. The funding allowed Liknaitzky to set up Australia's first university-based psychedelic research lab. It was groundbreaking stuff, but still he frequently butted up against stigma and taboo; he describes it as like 'cutting a path through the jungle'. Just getting his first delivery of psilocybin into the country in 2021 was a painstaking process that culminated in him being on the phone to the Australian

Border Force after they opened a strange package at Melbourne Airport and weren't sure it was all above board.

The Monash Clinical Psychedelic Lab quickly became a leading force in Australia's psychedelic research landscape. Within a year, Liknaitzky had pulled together a team of dozens of clinicians, and his earliest clinical explorations involved a world-first trial giving psychedelic therapists psilocybin as a way of helping them understand the experiences they would be overseeing in patients.

Among the many firsts that came out of the lab was his team's work with something called 5-MeO-DMT. Serving as an arm of a much larger international trial, Liknaitzky's team became the first ever in the country to use this drug in a clinical context.

THE MOUNT EVEREST OF PSYCHEDELICS

5-MeO-DMT is so structurally similar to DMT you'd be forgiven for thinking they were one and the same. But don't be mistaken. The effects of each drug are so profoundly different that you could say 5-MeO-DMT is about as similar to DMT as paracetamol is to heroin. And the story of 5-MeO-DMT plays out like a weird mirror to the 20th-century story of DMT.

Chemically, the drug has been recognised for a long time. A couple of Japanese chemists first synthesised it in 1939 and then, 20 years later, a couple of other chemists discovered the molecule in nature, in a humble South American bush called *Dictyoloma incanescens*.

In the 1960s a few pharmacologists catalogued the *possible* psychedelic effects of 5MeO in animal studies, but for the most part it remained a chemical footnote until a couple of influential moments near the end of the decade.

First, a team of anthropologists working among Amazonian

tribes looked into a psychedelic snuff. Investigating the resin, they discovered the main component was 5MeO.[18] Secondly, around the same time, an Italian pharmacologist named Vittorio Erspamer discovered high levels of 5MeO in the venom of an amphibian known as the Sonoran Desert toad.[19]

This information remained buried in dry chemical textbooks until a mysterious figure named Albert Most published an underground pamphlet in 1984 titled *Bufo Alvarius: The Psychedelic Toad of the Sonoran Desert*.* The tiny 18-page document described how to extract, prepare and smoke the toad venom. It spread through underground psychonaut circles and by the 1990s 5MeO was a certified psychedelic sensation.

The only real similarities 5MeO shares with its cousin DMT are that it cannot be metabolised through the gut. To get any effect, it must be smoked, snorted or injected. And, like DMT, it's short-acting. In and out – barely 20 minutes.

But the experience of 5MeO is nothing like DMT.

As mentioned, with DMT people often talk of being transported somewhere else. It can feel like being shot out of a cannon and across the universe only to land in a hallucinatory circus. The DMT space feels real, and it is so deeply detailed it must be somewhere else.

With 5MeO the experience is the exact opposite. Within seconds of imbibing it, a user is faced with absolute nothingness. It's sometimes described as a complete white-out. There are no hallucinations. There isn't even a sense of a 'self' experiencing things. It's an ineffable and vast blankness that many describe as terrifying.

---

* Psychedelic journalist and pharmacology researcher Hamilton Morris spent years trying to track down the real identity of Albert Most. He was eventually contacted by a man named Ken Nelson in 2019. Nelson claimed he was the real Albert Most and the author of the infamous *Bufo* pamphlet.

Think about it like this. Right now, if you look down, you will see your legs. Reach out and you will see your arms. The idea that your body is a vessel you are travelling around in can seem odd when you focus on it, but for the most part you filter away that embodied sense. With 5MeO, imagine your body disappearing – along with the world around it. Melting away in an instant. Leaving … what? Not even a 'you' is left to experience anything.

For some this experience of vast nothingness is exhilarating, blissful even. For others it is deeply frightening. Many scientists dub 5MeO the most potent psychedelic around, and Michael Pollan called it the 'Mount Everest of psychedelics', suggesting even hardened psychonauts approach it with caution.[20]

Perhaps one of the more interesting research pathways that has emerged in this 21st-century psychedelic renaissance is the clinical study of 5MeO as a treatment for depression. As big-money investors raced to snatch whatever psychedelic intellectual property they could, 5MeO and DMT both emerged as ideal short-acting candidates. But 5MeO unexpectedly took the lead.

As of 2026, there are two competing 5MeO medicines racing each other to the pharmaceutical-development finish line. One company, GH Research, developed an inhalable formulation of 5MeO; another company, AtaiBeckley, has a nasal-spray formulation. So the question must be asked: why has 5MeO dominated the research boom into short-acting psychedelics? Is it easier to utilise clinically compared to DMT? Is it more effective? Is it safer than DMT?

Very few of these questions have good answers right now. Maybe 5MeO is an easier substance to turn into a medicine compared to DMT? Sure, 5MeO gives users a potent white-out experience but when they return from their trip they are unlikely to be asking about the strange interdimensional elves. Maybe 5MeO is less ontologically challenging a drug for people to manage?

Not necessarily, according to Paul Liknaitzky. He and his Monash lab team played a notable role in the AtaiBeckley work, serving as a clinical trial site for their international 5MeO investigation. Liknaitzky has worked with a few different psychedelic medicines and suggests there are certainly clinical signs suggesting 5MeO is useful – for some people, at least.

But he does have some hesitations about its therapeutic utility. He sees the drug as so much more unpredictable than MDMA or psilocybin. It's also so deeply dissociative that from his perspective, as a psychologist, you have no idea what is going on in a patient's head while they are under its influence.

Liknaitzky likens the general practice of psychedelic medicine to strapping a patient to a rocket ship. Participants are given weeks of preparatory therapy. The training is there and the launchpad is set. When a drug is given, the rocket takes off. With some drugs, such as psilocybin, the therapist can act a little like ground control – helping the rocket to course-correct during take-off by triggering a side booster here and there when things start to go astray. But with 5MeO, his experience is that you are flying in the dark. You hit the big red launch button and whatever happens happens. The 5MeO experience is so fast, so powerful, so unlike anything else, that Liknaitzky wonders whether any therapeutic work can be done at all with it.

Contrasting the autobiographical experiences that can emerge with ayahuasca, 5MeO is not personal. Some participants in the trial Liknaitzky worked on found the experience of absolute dissolution helpful. In his words, it helped some people 'set up a kind of cosmic lantern of priority or value that then they can work toward in their lives'. However, not everyone felt that same way. And 5MeO's deeply weird nature left some participants merely confused – or, at best, bemused.

The drug may generate all those sought-after pharmacological effects modern drug developers are chasing. And maybe all those downstream neuroplastic effects are real and clinically meaningful. But is this the most effective, or even safest, way to get there?

Condensing the trip into a 10- or 20-minute mind blast may be the most cost-effective or scalable way to do psychedelic medicine. Sure. Pop into a clinic once or twice a year. Have a snort of this patented 5MeO nasal spray. Wash out the neural cobwebs, so to speak, and go home an hour later. It's the perfect way to integrate these drugs into our current 'move-'em-in and move-'em-out' medical system.

The thing I can't ever really get past, however, is how the broader philosophical impact of these drugs tends to be hand-waved away by modern drug developers. 5MeO may be physiologically safe. The drug certainly doesn't physically harm you. And psychologically it isn't necessarily dangerous. If we just track a number on a depression scale and show it improving after a dose, then we have a new medicine that works, right?

Except, as anyone with any type of personal experience with a psychedelic would immediately understand, it doesn't really work like that. Imagine your elderly mother. Never done a drug in her life. The biggest altered state she has ever encountered was the time she drank too many coffees in one day.

Her doctor prescribes her a 5MeO treatment. She pops into a day-procedure clinic for her little nasal puff, and bang – she encounters the most profoundly strange and discordant experience of her life. The mild depression she previously felt disappears. But the 5MeO experience has presented her with such a real, deeply felt sense of nothingness that she doesn't believe in God anymore. All her life she has been a devout Catholic, but now she has been to the end of the universe and seen that nothing is there.

How does a person return to their normal life after an experience like that? Your mother certainly can't go to her weekly church group anymore. Maybe she tries once or twice, but every time she goes, an argument about the existence of God comes up. Old friendships dissolve. Your mother isn't upset about this, though. She's on a new journey. And the shockwave of that single 5MeO trip ripples through your entire interpersonal family network.

This was just a small dose of medicine for her depression. But it changed everything.

Psychedelics can do this. And for some drug developers, this is not a feature of the treatment but a major bug that needs to be fixed. What if we could make a better medicine? A medicine that does all the useful anti-depression, anti-anxiety stuff but doesn't send someone to the outskirts of the universe leaving them questioning everything they thought was true and real about existence?

What if we can take the trip out of psychedelics?

TO TRIP OR NOT TO TRIP

During the first wave of research in the mid-20th century, psychedelic drugs were so deeply intertwined with psychiatry and psychotherapy that no one even considered there was a distinction between the trip and its accompanying mental health benefits.

As modern psychedelic clinical trials rolled out over the 2010s, however, a series of fundamental questions arose when scientists tried to investigate efficacy. How much of the benefit patients may get from psychedelics is due to the placebo effect? Is the antidepressant quality of psychedelics an artifact of the trip? Are people feeling a little better about their life because the psychedelic experience itself is shaking up their psychological world view?

One of the wildest experiments trying to tease apart these questions came in the early 2020s, when a team from Stanford

University looked at what happens when you give ketamine to patients while anesthetised for surgery. The fascinating trial recruited 40 patients with major depression who were planning to undergo simple elective surgery for some other medical condition.

While unconscious, half the cohort were given a 40-minute infusion of ketamine and half were given a similar infusion of saline. The experiment was perfectly primed to eliminate any bias – no need to worry about a placebo effect as both groups were asleep when given the drug. Over the days following the surgery, participants completed regular questionnaires measuring their depression symptoms.

The results, when published in 2023, proved profoundly controversial. The researchers found participants in both the ketamine and placebo groups showed similar improvements in depression scores. The findings contradicted a wealth of prior clinical trials testing ketamine for depression, all having consistently found the drug offered robust antidepressant effects.[21]

Could this be a sign that placebo response plays a major role in the well-documented antidepressant effects of ketamine? And what could this mean for psychedelic drugs, which confer an even more powerful subjective psychoactive experience? Could psychedelics be the ultimate placebo?

Like any single study, the findings were far from definitive. Lots of questions were lobbed at the researchers. Propofol, the primary anaesthetic drug used in the procedures, for example, has been suspected to have its own antidepressant qualities. Was the placebo group getting some kind of antidepressant benefit from *that* drug? Also, each participant was having their own unique surgical procedure during the trial, so there was no homogeneity among the cohort. Of course people would feel less depressed following a medical procedure if it improved a physical condition that was likely adding to their woes. Were people just feeling better because the surgery had worked?

Ultimately the study didn't really answer any questions but raised a whole batch of new ones. Perhaps most potently, a big question emerged: what does this mean for the pharmacological effect of classic psychedelics like DMT or psilocybin?

Since that landmark study the Stanford team has been slowly moving to perform the same kind of experiment with psilocybin instead of ketamine. And over in Switzerland another team of researchers is completing an even more direct trial: explicitly testing doses of DMT in patients with depression while under the effect of anaesthesia.

Regardless of any confounding issues, we'll have some more data soon on this issue. But let's speculate for a moment. What if we could re-engineer psychedelic drugs to remove *all* the hallucinatory effects? Would we be left with a whole new world of mental health medicines targeting specific brain receptors that could treat anything from depression and anxiety to addiction?

As cutting-edge advances in neuroscience uncovered some fascinating insights into how psychedelics do what they do in the brain, a collection of scientists began to work on taking the trip out of psychedelics. Their goal was simple: to create entirely new molecules that tickle specific brain receptors like psychedelics do, keeping their neuroplastic effects but getting rid of the psychoactive hallucinations.

HOW DO PSYCHEDELICS WORK? (AKA 'HANG IN THERE, WE'LL FIGURE THIS OUT TOGETHER')

Okay, so we've put this off for too long. In order to understand what psychedelics are doing in the brain, we need to talk a little bit of neurochemistry. I'll go easy on you; after all, I'm still figuring this out too.

Let's start with an oft-talked about molecule called serotonin.

It's the neurotransmitter responsible for a vast array of processes in the human body. Cognition, memory, appetite, sexual arousal, sleep: they are all in some way mediated by the ebbs and flows of serotonin. But the molecule doesn't just influence higher-order brain functions. You can find serotonin in all major organs in your body.

And it's not just a crucial molecule in humans. Serotonin is found in almost every living thing on Earth. It's virtually as old as life itself, with single-celled organisms developing serotonin billions of years ago as part of the photosynthesis process.[22]

As organisms evolved in complexity, so did their utilisations of serotonin. Jump forward to humans and we find a handsomely elaborate physiological system mediated by an intricate assortment of receptors, all tailored to be triggered by the molecule.

The chemical name we have given serotonin is 5-hydroxytryptamine (5-HT). Over the second half of the 20th century, scientists slowly discovered an unexpectedly broad array of receptors in the human central nervous system, all tuned to respond to serotonin. Turns out it's not just one receptor activated by serotonin. We now have now identified 14 different 5-HT receptors, spanning seven general classes.

Over the course of this book we've talked a lot about one particular 5-HT receptor: 5-HT2A (one of three different receptors in the 5-HT2 class). And there are good reasons for this. We know that the trademark characteristic 'trip' associated with psychedelics is fundamentally linked with the drugs' activation of these 5-HT2A receptors. We know this because when we give people psychedelics alongside drugs to specifically block the activation of 5-HT2A receptors, the subjective effects – the trip – of all classic psychedelics is also blocked.

You take a psychedelic like LSD or psilocybin, the molecule travels into the brain, clicks into these specific 5-HT2A receptors, and you start to trip? Is it as simple as that?

Well, not exactly.

As we've already seen, tiny differences in drug molecules (such as the minute difference between DMT and 5MeO-DMT) can result in earth-shatteringly divergent subjective experiences. And it's only recently that scientists have begun to understand just how many differing downstream effects can come from the activity of one kind of receptor.

For years researchers used the analogy of a lock and a key to explain how drugs interacted with various receptors. A receptor sat idle, like a locked door, waiting for the right molecule to come along. When that key floated by, it swiftly slipped into the lock, opening the door and activating everything that receptor was tuned to do.

But this binary 'on or off' idea has increasingly turned out to be the wrong analogy. Scientists know now that the downstream chain reaction of events triggered by any given receptor is deeply influenced by how a molecule *sits* in that receptor's binding site, known as the ligand binding site. So different molecules can slip into that receptor site and trigger varying effects.

All analogies are inevitably imprecise but think of this less like a lock and key and more like a hand in a glove. The natural hand that fits in a glove may have five fingers, but sometimes a hand with two, three or four fingers may slip into a glove. And when those irregular digits start wiggling around in the glove, unusual things can happen.

The neurotransmitter serotonin is the natural hand to the 5-HT2A receptor glove. But a variety of other molecules can also fit into that 5-HT2A glove, and each one wiggles in its own distinct way.

We also now know that not every drug that tickles 5-HT2A receptors causes subjective psychedelic effects in humans. It is possible to activate these receptors without generating a hallucinatory experience. And that also means it may be possible to create a novel molecule that slips into 5-HT2A receptors to generate antidepressant actions without causing psychedelic effects.

But things get a little more complicated, as we also now know that psychedelics don't *only* knock into 5-HT2A receptors. Turns out they do a remarkable assortment of other things in the brain. A massively rigorous study published in mid-2025 set out to catalogue exactly how many other receptors are hit by different psychedelic drugs. Forty-one different psychedelic molecules were tested and almost every one showed some level of binding to all 14 of the 5-HT receptors.[23]

Around 300 other receptors were studied and psychedelics were found to engage with a diverse array of mechanisms, from dopamine receptor processes linked to things like motivation, to adrenergic receptors, which play a role in hormonal regulation. These interactions affected everything from blood pressure regulation to physical alertness. Unsurprisingly, the study revealed pretty massive differences between psilocybin, LSD, mescaline and DMT when looking at what these molecularly similar drugs are doing in our brains.

While the findings of this truly landmark investigation amplified the head-spinning complexity of how psychedelics were likely influencing our brains and bodies, they did confirm one major hypothesis. The 5-HT2 class of receptor (A, B and C) was crucial to the psychedelic 'trip' part of these drugs. Researchers previously suspected the 'trip' was just 5-HT2A, but they were wrong. Despite all the other things going on with these drugs, the subjective nature of a psychedelic trip required tickling some combination of these three A, B and C receptors.

NOW, WE MAY HAVE SOME IDEA OF HOW THESE DRUGS generate their 'psychedelic' effects, but what kinds of ways could they be generating their therapeutic effects? Here, we need to dig a little deeper into an idea we have already briefly touched on: neuroplasticity.

Over the last 20 years, a compelling hypothesis has emerged in neuroscience. It attempts to present a neurobiological explanation for mood disorders such as depression.[24] The idea is that sustained levels of stress can cause neurons in the prefrontal cortex of the brain to atrophy. Similar to the way a muscle can slowly waste away when it is left unused, parts of the brain undergo structural changes that scientists suspect are associated with a variety of psychiatric conditions.

Picture a neuron in your brain like a bulb you might plant in the garden. Pretty quickly after planting, if the bulb is healthy, we should see lots of branches shooting out from it. In the context of a neuron, these branches are called dendrites, and in cases of depression we often see a retraction of spines from these dendrites. To reverse this process scientists look for compounds that promote what we call plasticity.

The first clue that certain drugs could do this came relatively recently. A study in 2010 was trying to understand what neurological process seemed to underpin the remarkably rapid antidepressant qualities of ketamine.[25] This new research in rats spectacularly demonstrated how ketamine stimulated the growth of dendritic spines in the prefrontal cortex within hours of dosing. Further work over the following years demonstrated ketamine producing increases in various other objectively measurable metrics like synaptic density and general neural excitability.

In 2018, a team led by American chemist and neuroscientist David E Olson coined the term 'psychoplastogen' to describe the growing family of small-molecule drugs that were found to promote these kinds of neuroplasticity.[26] Olson's work highlighted how certain psychedelics like LSD and DMT promoted dendritic spine growth in ways similar to ketamine. Over the following few years, drugs like psilocybin, 5MeO-DMT and MDMA were all found to affect neuroplasticity and sit under this new categorical banner of psychoplastogens.[27]

All of these extraordinary discoveries between 2015 and 2025 led to some wild propositions that researchers in the 1960s had never considered. Maybe the therapeutic effects of psychedelics could be divorced from the subjective hallucinatory qualities? Psychedelics are powerful drugs, that's for sure, but they're certainly not precision tools. In fact they are almost recklessly non-specific in the way they wash over our brains. They bump into so many different receptors and do so many different things that some researchers were bound to ask: what would happen if we started isolating really singular and targeted drug actions? Can we get plasticity without the trip?

THE NEW PSYCHEDELICS

'There's this saying that chemists come in two flavours: mild and wild. You can kind of pick each other. You get talking to people, things come up, and it's like a sort of coded language.'

Talking to Sam Banister, you'd never guess he was a wildly experienced medicinal chemist with a résumé that spans two decades of research. Instead he comes across as a contagiously enthusiastic psychonaut half his age (he's in his forties) who is keen to talk about everything from drugs and new molecules to the fundamentals of consciousness.

Like most involved in the modern psychedelic renaissance, Banister had long been interested in the potential of these drugs. During his undergrad degree, studying science in the early 2000s at the University of Sydney, he discovered the work of ethnobotanist Richard Schultes and his interests quickly moved to microbiology and botany. By the time he finished his PhD in 2011, Banister had completely fallen down the rabbit hole of medicinal chemistry. The idea of taking a molecule found in nature and tweaking it slightly to generate different psychoactive effects was his great interest, but at the time this research was as fringe as it gets in the academic world.

In 2014 he ended up immersed in the world of Californian science start-ups, embedding himself at Stanford. Studying alongside Nobel Prize–winning physiologist Brian Kobilka, who was exploring protein interactions with opioid and cannabinoid receptors, Banister learned exactly how new small-molecule drug development worked. Something was happening in the San Francisco Bay Area bubble and he could sense it: 'You have extremely straight, slightly autistic software-engineer friends who are saying, "I'm microdosing mushrooms for flow state and creativity,"' Banister recalls. 'And everyone you sit down next to in a cafe is a start-up founder of some sort.'

He ended up back in Australia by 2018 and wanted to go big with a moonshot: get a start-up company going here in Australia that focused on novel psychedelic chemistry. After a couple of years Banister met Josh Ismin, a Sydney-based founder. The two began to talk about the possibilities for some really serious drug development work in the psychedelic space.

When Covid hit, the pair got to building their new company – initially named Psylo but later rebranded to Xylo Bio. Armed with notebooks and laptops, they did all the initial groundwork for the company, like setting up bank accounts, while sitting in grassy parks between their homes, at the height of the pandemic restrictions.

The company initially had simple pragmatic goals, like maybe tweaking the psilocybin molecule to see if you could make a shorter-acting experience. But quickly Banister and Ismin saw other, bigger companies coming up with similar plans. There was no point playing catch-up with the big kids. If they were going to enter the space, their ideas needed to be bolder, further to the fringes.

Banister began to think back to the work he'd done in structural biology with other targets. Could they use super high-end computation, molecular modelling and virtual screening to discover entirely new areas of chemistry? Artificial intelligence systems can today scan millions of novel molecular combinations, test their receptor selectivity, and suggest potential new drugs at a speed never known in the past. So they forged ahead, with a focus on tweaking tryptamine molecules into new permutations.

TALKING TO SAM BANISTER ABOUT HIS VISION OF the future can quickly turn into a conversation that feels more sci-fi than science. The chasm between what we know in the public domain through published research journals and what is actually happening in start-up labs around the world is massive. Banister knows this because his Xylo journey is taking him to conferences all over the globe. Some are huge psychedelic conventions where the talk is big and the money even bigger. Others are smaller, niche pharmaceutical gatherings. Chemists come together to share their work, giving talks with titles so complicated that most of us would barely understand more than two words.

Before conference presentations, in the hallways outside lecture theatres, scientists inevitably chat about things they are doing – like new molecules they have discovered and are testing. Maybe some are even self-experimenting with these novel chemicals. These stories are not published in peer-reviewed journals, and they likely never will be, but they are happening.

Chemists are now teasing out different aspects of the psychedelic experience. Want to change the way you think about things but avoid the hallucinatory or perceptual disturbances that come with psychedelics? Someone is working on that. How about a new kind of MDMA experience that takes away the euphoric high but keeps the reflective therapeutic processes? That's in the works too.

A psychedelic experience is a broad confluence of many things. Some effects are purely sensory. Colours could seem brighter; music may sound different. Other effects are cognitive. You might think about things differently, connect two disparate ideas in ways you have never previously considered. In a psychedelic experience every neural input and output is altered to an uncanny degree. And with enough work, computational power and chemical innovation, Banister believes we could develop drugs with such specificity that single sensory processes are targeted.

THE TIP OF THE ICEBERG

Xylo has two big experimental molecules currently in development. The first is a new kind of antidepressant. This one is solely focused on stimulating 5-HT2A receptors and very little else. It's highly targeted, it's non-hallucinogenic, and early data on its antidepressant qualities in humans should be starting to leak out around 2027.

The second molecule is a little fancier. This one is described by Banister as a kind of balanced, non-hallucinogenic spin on psilocybin. Here they are targeting a few other receptors in combination with 5-HT2A, including 1A, 2B and 2C. It's their first genuinely bespoke new molecule. The clinical focus for this one is anxiety. If it works it will become a new kind of anti-anxiety drug – a non-addictive drug that gives you some of the long-term calming effects of psychedelics without the acute trip.

Xylo is one of a few companies around the world slowly starting to experiment with these new small-molecule drugs inspired by psychedelics. There's also another handful of scientists, working in academic surrounds, building up a broader body of knowledge. This is all incremental, piecemeal stuff. A tiny study here in a small chemistry journal on a niche receptor-binding event, and a tiny study there in an odd biology journal suggesting a small molecule has a certain effect on intracellular signalling.

By themselves these little bits of information mean very little, especially to anyone with zero interest in hardcore chemistry. But in totality they're the building blocks of a mind-bending future: a world in which we have hacked our neurochemistry to the point we can tweak our consciousness in whatever way we see fit.

BETTER LIVING THROUGH CHEMISTRY, MAYBE?

It's challenging to pull this whole conversation out of binary thinking, but every time I drilled down in conversation with someone about the 'trip or no-trip issue', we ended up in a grey area. Sam Banister was particularly keen to stress his frustration at the either/or positioning of the debate. As someone who is deep in the world of psychoplastogen development, he has no interest in eliminating the trip from all psychedelics. In fact, he's convinced there are already some clear therapeutic uses that seem entirely reliant on a patient having that full psychedelic experience.

'I would be shocked personally, and scientifically, if you could take a non-hallucinogenic agent for end-of-life anxiety, say, and have a dramatic reduction in anxiety scores immediately. I think a lot of that is tied to the psychological effects,' he tells me.

Banister hopes for a future in which a full spectrum of novel drugs emerges from this research – some, perhaps, are hallucinogenic, while others are less so. Maybe for certain conditions, fully psychedelic agents in combination with therapy will be necessary, but maybe a milder non-hallucinogenic psychoplastogen could be just as helpful for other people.

An analogy to SSRI antidepressants is particularly convincing. As Banister explains, our current antidepressant medicines are problematic drugs. They may help some people in times of crisis, but they have a torrent of side effects and are challenging to wean off.

If his new molecule work leads to a novel kind of antidepressant medicine with similar efficacy to current SSRI drugs but without the side effects, then that in itself would be a huge transformative event in mental healthcare. These drugs don't have to be magic bullets, Banister believes.

At the other end of the conversation, Paul Liknaitzky is sceptical the psychoplastogen work will do much more than maybe create a mild, new drug akin to SSRIs. That could be good, he notes, but it doesn't really get to the big life-changing movements that really help people. 'My sense is the value of psychedelics in being able to produce real and large and durable change in peoples' lives is because they facilitate very human experiences,' Liknaitzky argues. 'They can catalyse and amplify something that feels very real, often more real than ordinary awareness.'

At his core, Liknaitzky believes the big therapeutic benefits of psychedelics come from the way the drugs augment psychotherapy. A paper he co-authored in mid-2025 succinctly synthesised his attitudes on psychedelic medicines, and called for a complete change in perspective on psychedelic drug regulation. Subtitled 'Tools, Not Treatments', that article made a case for psychedelics primarily as adjuncts to psychotherapy.[28]

Using a clever comparison to anaesthetic drugs, the paper argued psychedelic research shouldn't be laser-focused on the paradigm of a drug treating a specific condition. Psychedelics, the authors reasoned, should instead be thought of as experiential medicines. Anaesthetic drugs, for example, are not treatments for specific conditions. Instead, they are used to induce a particular state that helps facilitate medical procedures. Liknaitzky argues we need to think about psychedelics in a similar way: as drugs that psychiatrists and psychologists can use to facilitate certain clinical outcomes.

At its core this idea certainly minimises the pharmacological impact of psychedelics, emphasising the big, mind-shifting changes that come with dramatic consciousness-changing experiences.

After more than a year of working on this book, and thinking about this one big question, I can only disappoint everyone by sitting on the fence. One part of me agrees with Liknaitzky. I mean, of course the enormous power of a psychedelic experience lies in the way it changes your mind so profoundly that every other day-to-day problem seems almost irrelevant. This is the gigantic ontological problem of psychedelic medicine. These drugs work because they change your mind, but they're also unpredictable and dangerous because they change your mind. Remember your elderly mum going in for that innocuous 5MeO-DMT treatment and coming out two hours later with a completely different perspective on God, the universe and everything?

But another part of me is wildly excited by Banister's speculations. The drug nerd inside me buys into the idea of better living through chemistry. In lots of ways it's simply a more sophisticated version of the world we already have. A world where we're constantly mediating our daily experiences with drugs. A dose of caffeine wakes up my brain in the morning. A dose of alcohol makes me more social. Maybe some THC helps me relax. Sugar gives me a mood boost.

Imagine a future in which we have so perfectly refined drug development that we can make a pill for anything. One pill makes you larger, and one pill makes you small ...

5

MDMA

HOW DOES THE THERAPY PART OF PSYCHEDELIC MEDICINE REALLY WORK?

'It can be challenging to be associated with what might be one of the meaningful experiences in a person's life. The scientist or clinician might, perhaps without explicit awareness, fall into the trap of playing guru or priest, imparting personal philosophies without a solid empirical basis ...'

Matthew W Johnson, 'Consciousness, Religion, and Gurus: Pitfalls of Psychedelic Medicine', *ACS Pharmacology & Translational Science*, 4(2), 2020, p. 580

In January 2024, a quietly momentous event took place in a small, innocuous Melbourne clinic. A patient was legally administered MDMA by an authorised psychiatrist for the first time in Western medical history. Of course, this wasn't the first time MDMA had been delivered clinically. Hundreds of patients had been given the drug in clinical trials. And several countries around the world had already started their own novel compassionate-use programs for various psychedelic drugs.[1]

But the dose in Melbourne that day was different. It was delivered by a psychiatrist, prescribed as a conventional medicine explicitly for post-traumatic stress disorder (PTSD). This followed Australia's historic regulatory shift in 2023, when the Therapeutic Goods Administration unexpectedly allowed MDMA to be administered as a treatment for PTSD and psilocybin for treatment-resistant depression.

Monica Schweickle, a clinical psychologist, was half of the dyad tasked with managing the session, alongside authorised psychiatrist Ted Cassidy. Due to a frustrating discordance in state-based regulations, the pair had to travel outside their home state of New South Wales to administer the treatment. (New South Wales had instituted a unique rule requiring psychedelic medicine to only be administered in hospital settings, but within a year the regulation was quietly removed from the state's rule books.)

So, very early that morning, Schweickle left her Melbourne hotel and went to the clinic to start getting things ready.

'I got to the clinic at 7 am – really early,' she reminisces, more than 18 months later. 'Tested all of the equipment, got all the food, made sure everything was perfect. I had a sense of anticipation. I wasn't nervous. I was really looking forward to it. It was exciting.'

It was Schweickle's first time supervising a psychedelic medicine session and everything went without a hitch. For the first hour or so, things were quiet in the dosing room as Schweickle and Cassidy sat with the patient. Then, suddenly, the patient became talkative.[2] Trauma experiences emerged, and as soon as the next day there was a real sense that progress had been made.

Two more MDMA dosing sessions over the following weeks were interspersed with integration therapy sessions. In a case study penned by Schweickle and Cassidy later in the year, they reported extraordinary results. One week after the second dosing session, the patient's PTSD score dropped to zero. And six months later it was still at zero. The patient's depression and anxiety scores also dropped to normal ranges by the end of the treatment, again remaining normal six months after finishing the treatment program.

'After the third dosing session, she began to feel comfortable leaving her children with their father or trusted family member to run errands for the first time,' the clinicians wrote in their case study. 'After the second dosing session [the patient] reported having greater self-compassion and being less troubled by the trauma memories. All these gains were maintained at three- and six-months post-treatment.'[3]

THE BLINDSIDE

Australia's Therapeutic Goods Administration (TGA) shocked many researchers and clinicians when it unexpectedly announced in early 2023 that it would be rescheduling MDMA and psilocybin.[4] The legislative shift created a new Schedule 8 entry for both drugs, which allowed them to be prescribed by authorised psychiatrists. The decision blindsided many experts in the field, seemingly coming out of the blue. Australia was generally known to be deeply conservative with its regulatory movements, so it was unusual to see it jumping so far ahead of the pack with psychedelic medicine.

The TGA's decision followed several years of expert consultation, on the back of extensive lobbying from a non-profit psychedelic advocacy group called Mind Medicine Australia.[5] Critics of the approval were concerned about the number of unresolved questions surrounding psychedelic medicines. Which patients would be best suited to the medicines? What were the best training methods for therapists? What kinds of psychotherapy should be used with psychedelics? How much psychotherapy would be necessary? No one even knew how long the benefits from the treatments would last. Nevertheless, Pandora's box had been thrust open and Australia was going to have to figure these things out as it went along.

Initially, things moved slowly. For the first six months after the new regulation switched on, not one patient was treated with either drug. By the beginning of 2026, two-and-a-half years in, fewer than 200 patients had been treated with MDMA or psilocybin, and around 60–70 psychiatrists had successfully applied to become authorised prescribers.[6]

To those concerned about the initial regulatory shift, this slow rollout was reassuring. However, no answers to any of those early questions had surfaced. Perhaps one of the most interesting and clear things to be seen in the early days of Australia's grand experiment was that MDMA seemed to be preferred by clinicians over psilocybin. Nearly twice as many patients had been treated with MDMA by early 2026 than with psilocybin.

After participating in more than 40 dosing sessions, Monica Schweickle had seen how useful MDMA could be and was not surprised it was being used more frequently. Psilocybin, and other classic psychedelics, can often incubate life-changing experiences. In fact, for many therapists, that transcendental mystical experience is what you want to generate, as it has been linked with a variety of beneficial therapeutic outcomes. However, as we have seen, alongside that kind of reality-shifting encounter comes a whole host of unforeseeable ontological consequences.

MDMA, on the other hand, is different. It is gentler. It floods one with a sense of comfort and sets the stage perfectly for frank psychotherapeutic interventions.

'MDMA is a good medicine to start with because it has a predictability that psilocybin doesn't,' Schweickle explains to me. 'I do love that about psilocybin: you never know what's going to happen, and have to prepare clients for that. But MDMA just has so much applicability to a whole range of human dilemmas – not just mental health treatments, but interpersonal and relational dilemmas.'

Schweickle isn't the only clinician working with these drugs to have expressed this sentiment to me. The impression I frequently get when talking to clinicians is that MDMA seems to be the ideal drug for modern therapy. In fact, if you were to design a drug specifically to facilitate effective psychotherapy, you probably would end up with something pretty similar to MDMA.

So, before we go any further, we need to ask some questions: what exactly is MDMA, and how is it so fundamentally different to the classic psychedelics we have been talking about so far?

IT'S NOT A CLASSIC PSYCHEDELIC DRUG

MDMA (or, to be specific, 3,4-Methylenedioxymethamphetamine) is a bit of a different drug compared to the psychedelics we have been talking about so far. Like classic psychedelics, MDMA interacts with a broad variety of receptors, including the whole 5-HT family. But the thing that makes this drug stand apart is that it's primarily what we call a serotonin–norepinephrine–dopamine releasing agent (SNDRA).

The main thing MDMA does when it enters your body is travel up to the brain and trigger a massive release of several key neurotransmitters, including the famous serotonin. This flood of chemicals throughout the brain and body leads to all the pro-social effects the drug is well known for: euphoria, happiness, connection to others, empathy.

The story of MDMA both precedes that of modern psychedelics and lives distinctly in its shadow. The chemical itself was first synthesised in Germany in 1912 by chemists working for the pharmaceutical company Merck. At the time it was just labelled a random intermediate chemical and not tested for any medical uses, and for the next few decades it sat in the dusty records of untested chemicals. Occasionally a chemist synthesised it and ran a couple of tests but it wasn't until the 1970s that its effects on humans were finally discovered.

The earliest human uses of MDMA are still shrouded in mystery. German researcher Torsten Passie spent several years tracing the history of the drug and his 2023 book *The History of MDMA* is perhaps the most exhaustive resource on how the drug spread in the 1970s and '80s.[7] The first traces of recreational use Passie detected were in 1970 when samples were reported by the Chicago Police Department, and more traces of the drug were identified by the authorities over the next couple of years.

It was around 1976 that MDMA came to the foreground for many researchers. Well-known American biochemist Alexander Shulgin had been experimenting on himself with new psychoactive molecules for years and, after hearing reports of the interesting effects of MDMA, he synthesised some and gave it a try. His early responses to the drug were surprisingly unenthusiastic. Shulgin famously described the effects of MDMA as akin to a 'low-calorie Martini' and reported nothing more exceptional than an 'alcohol-like intoxication'.

The very next year Shulgin met up with an old psychotherapist friend named Leo Zeff. Since the 1960s Zeff had been working with psychedelics therapeutically. As restrictions began to limit Zeff's use of drugs like LSD, he began working with a chemical called MDA. Zeff found the drug to be a useful adjunct to psychotherapy. It was more introspective than classic psychedelic drugs like psilocybin or LSD.

By 1977, Zeff was 65 years old and ready for retirement. A couple of years earlier he'd stopped using MDA therapeutically after a person in one of his group sessions suffered an unexpectedly toxic reaction. This side effect of MDA was becoming more well known, ultimately limiting its therapeutic uses. But Shulgin, suspecting possible interesting psychotherapeutic uses for MDMA, brought Zeff a parting gift. MDMA was less toxic than MDA, shorter-acting and more prosocial.

A few days later Shulgin's phone rang. Of course Zeff had tried the MDMA. And not only had he enjoyed the experience but he immediately put his retirement plans on hold. From that point forward Zeff became an evangelist for MDMA-assisted psychotherapy. Over the next few years he travelled across America and into Europe introducing psychotherapists to the drug. Informally, Zeff became known as 'the secret chief', mentoring hundreds of therapists while Shulgin kept him stocked with a constant supply of the drug.

If this MDMA therapy thing was so big in America, and parts of Europe, across the late 1970s and early 1980s, then surely there were some people doing the same thing in Australia? I put out a call through as many of my extended networks as I could, but hit dead end after dead end. I contacted Torsten Passie, the authority on the subject, and he had no knowledge of the drug being used therapeutically in Australia during this era. Every source I spoke to had no knowledge of the drug in Australia before the late 1980s. By then the drug was well established in its recreational capacity as 'ecstasy', and floating around nightclubs in most big Australian cities.

Then, in one random conversation, an interesting by-the-by footnote was dropped. Apparently, in a few Australian nightclubs circa 1987–88, MDMA distribution was allegedly connected to groups affiliated with the Rajneesh movement – a religious cult led by a guru known as Osho. Although still active today, despite the passing of its leader in 1990, the cult was most controversial for its activities in the United States across the early parts of the 1980s. I'd seen Netflix's *Wild Wild Country*. I was aware of the story of the 'Orange People', but this connection between the cult and MDMA was news to me.

Over in Australia, in the early 1980s, a very prominent Rajneesh community emerged in Fremantle, Western Australia. By 1984 the group numbered well over 400, and the Orange People were seen as an eccentric but accepted part of the local region. They ran a few restaurants and discos, and were known for their exuberant parties. With media reports beginning to recount stories of debauchery, violence and brainwashing, the group faced public pressure to move somewhere else.

As I tried to track down the earliest trace of MDMA use in Australia, sources told me that by 1985 the drug was indeed circulating through Rajneesh communities in Fremantle, and the police had started to notice. One of the first big MDMA busts in Australia was reportedly in a South Fremantle house populated by members of the Rajneesh community at some point in 1985–86. The date is unclear as the bust was not officially recorded as an illegal drug seizure because MDMA had not yet been formally scheduled in Australia. Lawyers working with the Rajneesh community managed to get all the charges dropped on that very basis. It simply wasn't illegal yet.

By the end of 1986, however, MDMA became, for all intents and purposes, illegal in Australia, and the next year the drug began to be tracked formally by law enforcement agencies and poison control databases around the country.

THE PERFECT DRUG?

In some ways, MDMA is the perfect drug for our modern times. It's a product of 20th-century chemistry, not found in any natural source. So there's no historical precedent of ceremonial or indigenous use. It doesn't deconstruct or dissolve one's sense of self in the same way as classic psychedelics. We have no fear of people taking MDMA and travelling to another dimension. There's no ontological shock, so to speak.

Instead, MDMA is the ideal accompaniment to a very modern kind of talk therapy – a type of therapy that centres trauma as the source of most mental health problems.

Today, a psychiatrist named Bessel van der Kolk is deeply influential in the world of modern MDMA therapy. His book *The Body Keeps the Score* has sold millions of copies since its first publication in 2014.[8] In it, van der Kolk presents a compelling hypothesis. He suggests repressed childhood trauma underlies almost all psychological and physical maladies. This simple idea underpins what is commonly known as trauma-informed care, an approach that assumes trauma is prevalent throughout society and works from the presumption that everyone has experienced trauma at some point in their life.

The implication is that past adversity explains current dysfunction, whether a patient realises it or not. If we accept that most of our ailments are the result of trauma, and accept that MDMA is an effective agent at precipitating trauma-based therapy, then it would make sense to see MDMA become commonly used, especially in comparison to other psychedelic medicines.[9]

In order to understand how MDMA is currently being used by clinicians both in Australia and around the world, we need to understand what kind of therapy is accompanying use of the drug. And we also need to understand how complicated things can get when you combine a drug that makes a person more open to new ideas with a psychotherapy intervention that is underpinned by powerful philosophical and spiritual beliefs.

In other words, if psychedelics enhance suggestibility, and some psychotherapies present powerfully specific world views, then we need to be very careful to understand the ethical stakes when patients engage with these novel treatments. It's not enough to simply ask 'Does MDMA-assisted psychotherapy work?' We need to ask *how* the therapeutic process could be influencing a person's inherent belief system.

DURING THE FIRST WAVE OF WESTERN PSYCHEDELIC medicine in the mid-20th century, American psychiatrist Sidney Cohen was at the forefront of some of the earliest LSD experiments. But by the end of the 1950s, he had started seeing red flags everywhere. He fell out with his long-standing research partner Betty Eisner, concerned she was falling prey to pseudoscientific ideas. Eisner had begun to believe patients were recounting experiences of past lives under the influence of psychedelics.

By 1960 psychedelic evangelism had reached fever pitch, and psychedelics were promoted in the media as a miracle cure for anything and everything. In his 1964 book *Beyond Within: The LSD Story*, Cohen expressed powerful concerns around the ways psychedelic drugs can supercharge a therapist's methods and influence a patient's outlook:

> It is curious how under LSD the fondest theories of the therapist are confirmed by his patient. Freudian symbols come out of the mouths of patients with Freudian analysts. Those who have Jungian therapists deal with the collective unconscious and with archetypal images. The patient senses the frame of reference to be employed, and his associations and dreams are molded to it ...
>
> Eventually the therapist becomes a highly significant figure to the patient. His notions of what is good and desirable tend to be adopted by the patient, and the therapist's overt or covert expressions of approval or disapproval come to constitute reward or punishment.[10]

Jump to the 2020s and we see eerie parallels in the boisterous psychedelic evangelism of advocates calling for the rapid and widespread use of these new medicines. The drugs have re-emerged into a distinctly specific and modern medical paradigm, and the hype is real.

In a milestone 2024 article about the ethics of modern psychedelic therapy, anthropologists Alex Gearin and Nicolas Langlitz point out the ecosystem of psychology in the 21st century is wildly diverse.[11] Psychiatric medicine today is very different to how it was in the 1960s. There are dozens of novel psychotherapeutic approaches and numerous psychoactive drugs being floated as useful.

'As the *form* of psychedelic-assisted psychotherapy experiences a renaissance, its *content* isn't what it used to be,' Gearin and Langlitz succinctly note in their article. 'Yet the many psychotherapeutic approaches that make up the psychotherapy component in psychedelic-assisted psychotherapy are not tested for safety or efficacy, only the drugs are.'

This thought sums up perhaps the biggest blind spot in our 21st-century psychedelic renaissance: how unexplored the therapy part of the process is. All clinical trial investigations of psychedelics have focused on simply comparing the drug with a placebo control. Trial protocols often wave the psychotherapy away without homing in on the specifics of what is happening in those sessions.

As a journalist covering this subject for several years, I've succumbed to this reductive oversimplification. I've written many stories on psychedelic medicine, and almost all of them have presented psychotherapy as a monolithic, uninterrogated process. I have written about the *importance* of psychotherapy, and I've written about how certain big pharma companies are trying to *reduce* its prominence in psychedelic medicine. But to date, there hasn't been one single study comparing the efficacy of psychedelics with different therapy modalities. What is the most effective type of psychotherapy to pair with psychedelics? Would it surprise you if I told you that no one knows – or that, possibly, it doesn't even matter?

'Much to our surprise,' Gearin and Langlitz noted in their 2024 article, 'most of the psychedelic therapists we interviewed felt that the specific modality of psychotherapy was not all that important.' A meta-study of psychotherapies published in 2017 came to a similar conclusion. The analysis was gigantic; it looked at around 500 different clinical trials that tested various psychotherapies for depression over 40 years. And the conclusion? 'Several different types of psychotherapy have been developed and tested. All have been found to be effective compared with waiting list, care-as-usual, and placebo control conditions.'[12]

So maybe it simply doesn't matter what kind of therapy accompanies psychedelic medicine? The elements often cited as most important to a treatment's success transcend particular modalities; they tend to be about the bond between a therapist and patient, and the authenticity of the therapist.

'I'M NOT A PSYCHONAUT'

For nearly 20 years, Sydney therapist Ariana Elias has focused her clinical work on how best to treat patients suffering from severe eating disorders, and for most of that time she's been determinedly agnostic about different schools of psychotherapy. Whatever she can adapt to help her patients has been the goal. She has trained in everything she can: cognitive behaviour therapy (CBT, and CBT-E), trauma-focused CBT, dialectical behaviour therapy (DBT), specialist supportive clinical management (SSCM), family-based treatment (FBT), internal family systems (IFS) and deep brain reorienting (DBR).

Elias knew there was no single magic bullet to be found. But her ever-growing toolbox of techniques helped her treat more and more patients. 'As the years went on I sort of started getting to what seemed to be an exhaustive list of therapies, and I was still finding there was at least a section of people in the eating disorder space that weren't responding. Then, in 2020, I came across ketamine,' Elias tells me.

Ketamine was Elias's first encounter with a drug-assisted psychotherapy. At the time the drug was mostly being used for either depression or trauma therapy. Recognising how intertwined those problems were with eating disorders, Elias jumped at the opportunity to head overseas and train in a new treatment modality.

'I knew nothing about psychedelics,' she tells me. 'I'm not a psychonaut. I never used psychedelics as a kid, as an adolescent, as a young adult. So it was, again, something completely new and foreign to me. I couldn't find very much on its application with eating disorders, but I started thinking about whether it could have any utility in the eating disorder space.' She was soon drawn into the world of psychedelic medicine, and founded a ketamine-assisted therapy clinic in Sydney when she returned to Australia.

MDMA was another drug that caught her eye. As a drug that was seemingly working amazingly for PTSD, she was keen to get trained and begin to see if it could help her patients.

In the early 2020s the main MDMA therapy training was done by Rick Doblin's MAPS organisation. MAPS was the big non-profit company pushing MDMA for PTSD research. At the time the work was deep into Phase 3 clinical trials and MAPS frequently ran therapist-training programs.

Again, Elias had to travel overseas for the training. And in a moment of unexpected synchronicity, she returned to the country ready to get to work just as the TGA was announcing its landmark regulatory changes. So, using the MAPS model, Elias got to work exploring the potential of MDMA-assisted therapy in her most treatment-resistant eating disorder clients.

> We used the MAPS model training protocol. We used a lot of very focused inner healing intelligence in the room. It was a trauma-focused model so I was looking for trauma. What I found, which was really so interesting, is that absolutely trauma emerged. These patients were completely blown away and shocked at connecting with this past trauma that they hadn't realised they'd been connected to in all the years of treatment.

In the chats I had with Ariana, the process of how MDMA therapy worked really jumped out at me. MDMA seemed to bring about memories of traumatic events that patients had been unable to connect with previously. And, in confronting those memories, patients are told to rely on something called their 'inner healing intelligence' to help process these experiences.

So is MDMA therapy about recovering forgotten traumatic memories?

THE MEDICINE TELLS YOU WHAT YOU NEED TO KNOW

'I think it is helpful to remember nothing is going to come up that is not already there,' explains a model therapist to a patient in a role-play scenario laid out in MAPS' treatment guide for therapists, *A Manual for MDMA-Assisted Psychotherapy in the Treatment of Posttraumatic Stress Disorder*. The role play is shown as an example of how a therapist could respond to a patient who was concerned about memories that may emerge during an MDMA dose session.

The therapist continues:

> Whatever comes up is something you are walking around with already but maybe not fully conscious of. I know it can be scary. The paradox is, although this approach could stir up memories or even flashbacks, temporarily, it allows you to move through them in a way, so that you are actually more apt to be free of them and less likely to have them be a problem for you in the long run. It's possible you could have more symptoms temporarily, like we talked about.[13]

The idea that MDMA therapy can restore lost traumatic childhood memories is far from a niche or academic concept. In fact, one of the most popular depictions of modern MDMA therapy in recent times was entirely concentrated around this process. In early 2025, Amy Griffin published a memoir titled *The Tell*. It was a blockbuster, spending a month on The New York Times Best Sellers list and selling over 100 000 copies. Oprah Winfrey chose it as a Book Club Pick and Griffin embarked on a star-studded book tour across the United States, along the way becoming one of *Time* magazine's most influential people of the year.

The book recounted Griffin's life story, a life that from the outside seemed perfect. She was rich and successful; everything appeared normal. But her behaviour as an adult grew increasingly erratic. She was racing through life, snapping aggressively at minor frustrations. She wasn't happy.

Griffin's husband, John, was a billionaire hedge fund investor. He donated money to the MAPS research fund (a fact not disclosed in Amy Griffin's book). Sometime after John's million-dollar donation, he began doing MDMA therapy with an underground guide. Noticing his wife's inner discomfort, he suggested she meet his therapist, Olivia, who had been connected to the Griffins informally via Rick Doblin, the founder of MAPS. At dinner, Olivia explained she isn't really a therapist – more a facilitator.

And here Griffin began her journey with MDMA therapy.

'The day of the session, I was anxious. "There's something I can't face," I told Olivia. "I know something happened to me, something I'm talking around. But I don't know what it is. It's like I can't remember. Or maybe I don't want to remember."'[14]

Five minutes into Griffin's first MDMA session, a memory flashed back with extreme vividness. She described it like a film playing inside her head. Her adult self watched as her younger self was violently raped by a teacher that she'd thought was 'one of the good ones'. Over the course of two more MDMA sessions, Griffin's memories got more and more detailed. She wrote of this teacher sexually assaulting her several more times over the next few years.

The book is an undeniably powerful read, recounting a kind of liberation story. Griffin overcomes her buried trauma and transcends the constraints of perfection after being shackled by a patriarchal society. It's confronting but also inspirational, and unsurprising in its popularity.

A few months after *The Tell* was published, however,

the elephant in the room emerged. A rigorously researched *New York Times* article was published interrogating the veracity of the forgotten trauma memories Griffin had so richly described.[15] Much of the latter part of Griffin's book follows her journey trying to figure out what actually happened, and while the story does end with a figurative question mark as to the presence of objective proof, there is never any doubt expressed in the book that these were real memories.

The *New York Times* journalists interviewed dozens of people in the course of reporting the story – from residents in Griffin's hometown to the local law enforcement officials who actually investigated her claims. Interviewees were uniformly surprised that this particular teacher was linked to such violent abuse. In the months following the publishing of the book, local police braced themselves for more victims to come forward.

A detective in the local Special Victims Unit expressed surprise that no other victims could be found. 'They don't stop,' he told reporters. 'I've worked older cases before. You find other people.'[16]

Yet no other victims emerged.

ARIANA ELIAS HAS SEEN PATIENTS EXPERIENCE profound healing and growth after having extraordinarily upsetting memories surface during drug sessions. Her thoughts echo those of several other psychedelic therapy practitioners I have spoken to. There seems little doubt of the healing power in unearthing traumatic memories during MDMA therapy.

But what of the veracity of those emerging memories?

'I don't think it matters if what they're telling us is the truth in its entirety,' Elias explains frankly. 'It's enough if it's *their* truth. And I feel very, very comfortable just being with whatever comes up for them and working with whatever that is, with the goal and purpose of helping them heal from it, rather than it becoming all about how specific and detailed it is.'

The trauma Elias hears about can be 'catastrophic, really catastrophic', she says. 'We're talking about incest, paedophilia, the most horrendous of horrendous crimes. But these patients are not trying to press charges against people. They're actually just trying to heal. So, how exact the detail of the memory is, for me, less relevant, and what's more relevant is just being with them and supporting them to have language to share what's trapped in their body so that we can heal.'

The story of Evelyn Harrison, recounted earlier in this book, is a similar one of extraordinary liberation and healing stemming from the recovery of a lost childhood trauma memory. Evelyn's description of the way she felt a weight release after experiencing the recovered memory is impossible to ignore. However, among all the other stories of early psychedelic therapy I came across, the account from Vivien Achia in 1960s Melbourne stood in powerful contrast (see Chapter 1).

Vivien's story also tells of the emergence of a lost memory during psychedelic therapy. Except for Vivien, the memory could not have happened. For reasons of privacy Vivien has asked that certain details of her story remain private, but what I can disclose is the memories of abuse that emerged for her were not by an anonymous figure. She resisted the clinicians at Newhaven hospital who were pressing her to accept these memories as real, because she knew that if she were to assume they were fact, they would cause irreparable fissures in her large social and familial networks.

For Evelyn, believing the memory led to little interpersonal friction. Her abuse had come from a random, anonymous figure in a park when she was young. Accept the memory, integrate it, and heal. For Vivien, it was far from that simple.

In Amy Griffin's bestselling memoir, her abuser is ostensibly kept anonymous, but in reality, everyone in her small town quickly put the pieces together and figured out who she was referring to. The *New York Times* journalists attempted to track him down in their reporting but they couldn't find him. Locals suggested the teacher had not been seen since the book was published.

Separate to any possible legal outcomes that could arise from these drug-assisted recovered memories, the social shockwave through a community is impossible to understate. With MDMA therapy we see the acceptance of a new therapeutic paradigm that fundamentally believes in the truth of recovered memories, and this is not something that can be taken lightly.

Particularly since this is far from a new idea.

The idea that psychedelics help treat mental illness by unlocking repressed memories surprisingly goes all the way back to their initial uses in Western medicine during the first wave of psychedelic psychiatry. One of the earliest published reports of LSD-assisted psychotherapy in 1950 explicitly points to the drug being useful in helping patients 'remember and relive' childhood experiences.[17]

UK psychiatrist Ronald Sandison most explicitly laid out this framework for psychedelic psychotherapy in his 1954 article 'The Therapeutic Value of Lysergic Acid Diethylamide in Mental Illness'.[18] Here Sandison described the 'recovery of repressed childhood memories' as of 'utmost importance' to the therapeutic value of the treatment.

For Sandison, an advocate of Carl Jung's ideas, the veracity of any memories recovered was never in question. In fact, despite the field of psychiatry in the 1950s being distinctly split between Freudians and Jungians, both schools of thought agreed with the fundamental idea of our unconscious suppressing certain memories. And psychedelics quickly became a useful tool in unlocking those buried experiences.

When psychedelic medicine moved out of general practice, the idea of psychoanalysis recovering lost childhood memories hung around. And in the early 1980s a considerable controversy bubbled to the surface.

SATAN AND THE MEMORY WARS

Canadian psychiatrist Lawrence Pazdar had been working with Michelle Smith for three years when he got the call that his long-time patient had been hospitalised after a severely traumatic miscarriage. The failed pregnancy seemed to have awoken something in Smith, and after half a dozen visits following the trauma she expressed an unexpected thought to Pazdar.

'There's still something bothering me,' she said. 'I still feel blocked. We talk about the things I *think* are the problems, and then I go home and spend half the night … wishing I could. … I know there's something I want to tell you, but I don't know what it is!'[19]

As recounted in the book the pair subsequently wrote, *Michelle Remembers,* Pazdar and Smith spent the next 14 months excavating those lost memories. What emerged was nothing short of astounding: a tale of ritualistic abuse at the hands of a satanic cult in the 1950s when Smith was just five years old. From human sacrifices to torture and sexual assault, the book luridly immersed itself in the unfolding memories.

The idea of recovered memories had crashed into mainstream pop culture. A wave of similar cases quickly emerged, leading to what was later dubbed the 'satanic panic' – a kind of collective hysteria that swept the United States. By the early 1990s more than 12 000 cases of satanic ritualistic child abuse had been reported. Come 1994 the panic had receded, and not one of those 12 000 cases was ever substantiated.[20]

A battle had broken out in the world of psychology and psychiatry. Essayist Frederick Crews called the skirmish the 'memory wars', using it as the title of his 1995 book.[21] The fight was fierce – between those who believed in the veracity of recovered-memory therapy and those who thought false memories were being created. And the stories emerging weren't just wild satanic rituals. Using a variety of therapeutic techniques, including hypnosis, people were reporting profound stories of childhood abuse, incest and paedophilia.

Some of these cases inevitably ended up in legal proceedings, and psychologists appeared in court to represent both sides of the argument. The most prominent figure in the false memory camp was a psychologist named Elizabeth Loftus. Appearing as expert witness in a variety of high-profile cases, her 1994 book *The Myth of Repressed Memory* became a defining text in the story of the memory wars.[22] On the other side of the fence was Bessel van der Kolk, who attempted to present a neurobiological argument for how the brain can repress memories.

In the end, the memory wars were never fully resolved. Loftus and her side perhaps came out of the ruckus on top. The extremity of the satanic memories led most scientists to discredit the idea of repressed memories as an unreal, or at least *unreliable*, phenomenon.

But those practising these therapeutic modalities didn't disappear. They were still around, albeit temporarily pushed to the fringes of clinical credibility. And in Australia the true repressed memory believers found a way to dominate the public conversation as the new millennium got underway.

CATHY KEZELMAN AND THE CLOAKS

In the late 1990s Cathy Kezelman was a successful GP with a thriving practice in Sydney. She had a loving husband and was mother to four energetic children. When her niece died unexpectedly in a car accident, Kezelman's world abruptly fractured. She fell into a depression and after a few months made the decision to see a psychologist.

After a few weeks her therapist raised the topic of childhood, and Kezelman quickly discovered she was missing large chunks of her earliest memories.

In 2010 Kezelman published a memoir titled *Innocence Revisited*.[23] The book spanned nearly a decade of therapy in which Kezelman progressively recovered more memories of her childhood, and those memories became more and more horrific. Beginning with sexual assaults being perpetuated by a family doctor, the recovered memories shifted to recurring violent rapes by her father, sometimes even at gunpoint.

Kezelman's book, and her therapeutic journey, culminated in a series of richly described, utterly harrowing sequences in which she was subjected to satanic rituals by a cult-like group who wore hoods and gathered in a cave somewhere near a beach in Sydney. Kezelman ultimately recovered memories of watching a young girl being dismembered on a stone altar by a group she referred to as the 'Cloaks'.

At the time Kezelman was recovering all these traumatic memories, she was chair of an organisation called ASCA (Adults Surviving Child Abuse). Following the publication of *Innocence Revisited,* Kezelman became a prominent figure in formulating Australia's broader policies around childhood trauma and abuse. She received an Order of Australia medal in 2015, and then rebranded ASCA as the Blue Knot Foundation in 2016, subsequently receiving millions of dollars in government funding to establish training and support systems for both psychologists and survivors of childhood abuse.

In 2017, Kezelman's brother broke his silence to publicly refute all the stories in *Innocence Revisited*. He claimed the extreme memories of satanic abuse or rape by gunpoint could not have happened.[24]

Despite the unusual echoes of satanic panic stories in Kezelman's memoir, I was struck by how deeply the paradigm of recovered trauma memories was embedded in modern Australian psychology literature. In the late 2010s Kezelman's Blue Knot Foundation published several key practice documents describing foundational ideas behind what is now known as 'trauma-informed' therapeutic practice.

One of those documents in particular discusses memory and the idea of recovered memory. The 48-page report serves as a kind of defensive case for the veracity of recovered trauma memories.[25] In a world where the scientific community is still very much debating these ideas, I read the report as uncomfortably one-sided.

After spending months investigating this fraught debate around recovered trauma memory, I came away with a sense of uneasiness. I offer no opinion as to the veracity of anyone's experience of recovering forgotten trauma memories. But what did seem to me like a looming problem was the way these therapeutic processes could be supercharged by the addition of psychoactive drugs such as MDMA.

WITH THE RENAISSANCE OF MEDICAL PSYCHEDELICS, the recovered-memory true believers re-emerged, stronger and with a whole new set of foundational texts. Not everyone doing MDMA therapy in Australia is working within this recovered-memory paradigm, but it not only is common, it's implicitly imprinted into the most popular psychedelic therapy training protocol in the world. Practitioners I spoke to, both on and off the record, discussed a number of patient experiences in current, legal MDMA therapy involving recovering forgotten traumatic memories.

Ariana Elias, for example, candidly told me about two successful recent patient experiences she guided that both centred around the emergence of forgotten memories. She suggested the patients both independently verified the truth of the recovered memories but those investigations were not directed by her. In fact, Elias told me the truth of the memories that emerged in her patients wasn't of great concern. 'In the end, I don't know that it matters.'

Monica Schweickle echoed this sentiment, telling me the story of a patient who completed a three-dose course of MDMA therapy focused on PTSD that was thought to be associated with a single work-related incident. His initial therapeutic course was successful, with huge reductions in all his PTSD markers. But it seemed like the MDMA therapy unlocked something, and Schweickle's subsequent (non-MDMA) sessions with him are now uncovering more and more repressed trauma memories.

'Each time we meet for a session, he's got a new trauma memory,' Schweickle told me. 'And they're getting earlier and earlier.'

The technique Schweickle uses, called EMDR (eye movement desensitisation and reprocessing) was developed in the late 1980s.[26] It involves invoking parts of traumatic memories while engaging in specific types of somatic stimulation, such as left-to-right eye movements or finger tapping. Exactly how EMDR works is still unclear but a number of clinical trials have shown it to be an effective treatment for PTSD.

For Schweickle and her patient, each consecutive session helps to reprocess these newly recovered trauma memories. She describes it as like a process of digging through different buried layers, at the patient's own pace. What was thought to be PTSD due to a single incident turned out to be a severe and complex trauma that went all the way back to the patient's youngest years.

'THIS CAN'T BE THE STARTING POINT'

Kayla Greenstien has always been sensitive to the dynamics of cult brainwashing. After all, she grew up in a cult herself.

Just south of Vancouver, Canada, in a small suburban farming community, Greenstien's dad was part of a group known as the Worldwide Church of God. Her parents were classic middle-class, '80s baby boomers with a distinct penchant for New Age and fringe beliefs.

Instinctually, and perhaps rebelliously, she had a deep aversion to the religious atmosphere that suffocated her home life. By the age of 13 she had already been expelled from one school and spent time in a psychiatric hospital. A trip to visit relatives in Japan the following year showed her there could be a way out. Education was her escape – and then, in her first year of university, she discovered psychedelics.

It was amazing, life-changing, but her aversion to New Age groupthink kept her on the periphery of the traditional 'Burning Man' psychedelic community. She bounced around the world for a few years: France, Toronto, Vietnam, and finally Australia. Her psychology studies led to her working in a rape crisis centre while she finished her degree.

In early 2021 a colleague mentioned to her the growing work going on with psychedelics and psychotherapy. It was all new to Greenstien. She'd had her own profoundly meaningful experiences with psychedelics, but she had not at all been paying attention to the burgeoning research. 'I hadn't even read the Michael Pollan book,' she exclaimed to me. 'I was pretty disconnected from it all.'

In Australia, at the time, there was one main psychedelic therapy training program so Greenstien signed up for it. 'I make a lot of decisions very rashly, and I was like, "All right. Let's go. Let's do this."'

The course started in the Covid universe of July 2021, and the first wave of sessions was all online. Considering the serious way the course was presented, accompanied by dozens of big-name-psychiatrist recommendations, Greenstien was expecting a rigorous, science-heavy experience. But pretty quickly she started picking up some 'weird vibes'. A few people in the training course began quietly raising issues during the Zoom sessions.

One video the cohort watched, for example, depicted a few clinicians role-playing a dosing session. To explain how one goes about gaining consent from a patient regarding the use of touch, the therapist asks, 'Is it okay if I touch you?' – literally as he puts his hand on the patient.

'And that was the entire consent process,' Greenstien tells me with a still-fierce sense of exasperation. 'After their role play, one of the psychiatrists [participating in the training] said, "I'm sorry but you can't ask for consent while touching someone." She raised it as a real issue.'

This was the beginning of a chain of problems that seemed to continually emerge, and for Greenstien things reached a surreal point in September 2021 when one of the first big psychedelic medicine scandals hit the news. Two of the most well-known international trainers of new psychedelic therapists had been accused of misconduct by several former patients.

Aharon Grossbard and Francoise Bourzat had been practising psychedelic therapy in an underground context for more than two decades. The husband-and-wife pair had taken a prominent role in the dawning psychedelic renaissance, playing a part in many therapy training programs around the world. But a former patient named Will Hall broke his silence, accusing the pair of alleged misconduct and violating professional boundaries.[27] Pretty soon after Hall's allegations emerged, more former patients came out to recount their experiences of abuse and inappropriate behaviour. Journalist Katie MacBride's investigations into the matter subsequently revealed seven more sources corroborating the misconduct.[28]

Grossbard and Bourzat have consistently denied all allegations of inappropriate conduct.

These reports came out literally one week after Francoise Bourzat had given a presentation to Greenstien's training cohort. So, being the firebrand she is, Greenstien started sending emails to the people running the training program.

'I remember [one response] to me very clearly: "I just like to focus on the good work going on." And I was like, "What the fuck kind of response is that?"' Greenstien recalls. 'This is where I realised, "Something really wrong is going on here."'

Coming out of working at a rape crisis centre, where she had seen many cases of institutional cover-up following this exact same pattern, Greenstien was furious, and a little stunned: 'This can't be the starting point. This *cannot* be the starting point.'

With her critical radar pinging, Greenstien started digging into the training program's coursework. Here, she came across a bunch of ideas she could only interpret as 'weird'. Holotropic breathwork, a technique involving fast breathing leading to altered states of consciousness, and inner healing intelligence were two of the biggest ones that quickly jumped out at her as unconventional.[29] What was being presented as 'scientific' and 'evidence-based' certainly didn't feel that way.

She, and several others, quickly pulled out of the training program.

Greenstien had previously been working on a nascent PhD

looking at psilocybin as a treatment for complex PTSD, but now her focus dramatically shifted. Her work today investigates the ethics of touch in psychedelic therapy.

Francoise Bourzat continues to teach psychedelic therapy training programs around the world. As of early 2026, she was still teaching prominently in the same Australian psychedelic therapist training course Greenstien dropped out of.

Greenstien certainly wasn't the first person I had talked to who brought up the idea of inner healing intelligence. It seemed to be deeply entrenched in modern MDMA therapy, and the more I investigated, the more it reminded me of a longstanding New Age belief that I had bumped up against several times in my youth.

CHANGE YOUR MIND, CURE YOUR SELF

I was in my mid-twenties, standing in the kitchen of a share house just talking junk with my housemate. We were all different shades of hippy so I guess my housemate felt it was a safe space to start espousing on the philosophy of someone named Louise Hay. This was the first time I had heard of Hay, and my instinctual response was not kind.

'All physical disease stems from emotional disturbances,' my housemate proclaimed. You see, he told me, psychological root causes manifest in physical symptoms. And what's more, by 'changing your mind', so to speak, you can cure your physical illness.

'Hang on,' I interjected. 'What about children? Babies born with chronic illnesses? You're saying it's their fault they are sick?'

A nerve had been touched. And to be fair, my housemate was entirely unaware that I had been struck with a chronic autoimmune condition in my younger years. So it was a sensitive subject for me. But I suspect that wouldn't have changed the tenor of the conversation.

'Babies absorb the emotional energy of their parents,' she countered. 'Disease in the young is a manifestation of negative environmental energy. Affirmations can help healing.'

I can't remember exactly how this interaction ended. I likely ended up angry, feeling like this entire belief system fundamentally blamed the individual for being sick. And I took it personally. Was it my fault for getting seriously ill when I was 12? Was my still-chronic illness the result of negative energy projected on me from my parents? Did I remain seriously unwell for the better part of a decade because I simply never changed my mind effectively?

In the years following I learned more about Louise Hay. I discovered she was one of the biggest-selling non-fiction authors on the planet. And she made a career out of telling people they can heal themselves, and that no illness could be separated from a person's inner-emotional world. In fact, Hay had specific, prescriptive affirmations for almost any physical disease you could face.

Cancer? That's caused by longstanding resentment. Maybe a deep secret or grief eating away at the self. Thyroid problems? That's humiliation. Had a miscarriage? You likely harbour a deep fear of the future.

I guess for some people the idea that 'you can heal yourself' is liberating. It gives one a sense of control over the sometimes-chaotic randomness of life. That feeling is likely powerful … for some. But to me, someone who was struck with a chronic illness when very young, possibly from multifaceted genetic and environmental causes, this way of thinking made me feel like it was *my fault* I got sick. And that it was my fault I was still sick.

But it's not my fault I was sick. And it's not my fault I still am sick. We can't heal ourselves just by thinking positively and reciting some daily affirmations. I *didn't* believe that. I *couldn't* believe that. And if we are to establish any kind of medical system based on evidence and science, I simply *wouldn't* believe that.

Years later, when I learned about the idea of inner healing – an idea that seemed to be the foundation of modern MDMA-assisted psychotherapy – my personal sceptic radar pinged. Being a journalist, however, I work hard to recognise my prejudices. And so I withheld any knee-jerk judgment. I wanted to talk to the experts to try and understand things.

Okay ... what is this whole 'inner healing intelligence' thing all about?

ALMOST EVERY ABOVE-GROUND MDMA THERAPY practitioner working today utilises, in some way, the therapy manual developed by MAPS.[30] The manual was developed as a way of providing a consistent therapeutic model unifying the many clinical trial sites around the world as research progressed testing MDMA for PTSD. Now, it serves as the backbone for many psychedelic therapist training programs.

Many MDMA therapists I spoke to in the process of researching this book mentioned deploying some form of inner healing process in the context of working with the drug. The language each therapist used varied. Some didn't like the phrase 'inner healing intelligence' and played around with the nomenclature, but the general idea of inner healing being an important facet of the treatment was consistent.

As described in the MAPS manual, the concept of inner healing intelligence is based on the idea that true healing is an innate process that resides inside every patient. To encourage patients to trust in their own inner healing intelligence, the manual suggests a therapist might explain the concept by saying: 'We encourage you to approach whatever comes up as something that's coming up as part of your healing process. We trust that your inner healing intelligence will bring you what you need for healing and that's much more reliable than anything you or we could figure out ahead of time with our rational minds.'[31]

Whatever experience or memory that emerges during a MDMA dosing session, the patient 'should be encouraged to cultivate an attitude of trust in the wisdom and timing of the inner healing process that is catalyzed by this approach', according to the manual.[32]

The treatment is presented, ostensibly, as non-directive. The therapist is often referred to in the manual as a 'guide', whose role is to 'remind the participant that facing painful experiences is actually a path toward healing'.[33]

And if you are still a little unclear on how inner healing intelligence works, the MAPS manual offers this analogy to help therapists explain the concept to patients:

> The body knows how to heal itself. If someone goes to the emergency room with a laceration, a doctor can remove obstacles to healing (e.g. remove foreign bodies, infection, etc.) and can help create favorable conditions for healing (e.g. sew the edges of the wound close together), but the doctor does not direct or cause the healing that ensues. The body initiates a remarkably complex and sophisticated healing process and always spontaneously attempts to move toward healing. The psyche too exhibits an innate healing intelligence and capacity.[34]

The idea certainly *feels* like it makes sense. After all, the body kind of does heal itself, when you think about it. But the analogy swiftly falls apart when you consider the importance of human intervention in *helping* the body heal itself.

A doctor may not be causing the healing of a broken bone, but some breaks aren't repairing themselves without significant third-party interventions, such as bones being reset or even surgically pinned. And that infection isn't going to go away by itself either. Sometimes antibiotics are the difference between life and death.

The body may be able to heal itself, but it often needs lots of help. And that 'help' is basically the definition of all modern medicine.

But where does this idea of inner healing intelligence come from? As one MDMA researcher said to me, this is not an empirically supported idea and it's not particularly coherent: 'Why would MDMA show people what they need to experience?'

Well, it all goes back to a psychiatrist named Stanislav Grof.

THE GROF OF IT ALL

Stan Grof was a big player in exploring the therapeutic potential of LSD in Prague during the 1950s and '60s. Unsurprisingly, he ended up in the United States by the late 1960s. Following the general prohibition on psychedelic research, Grof worked as part of the only legal LSD investigation in the US, at Spring Grove hospital in Maryland. Those studies continued until around 1976; however, Grof had left for the sunny shores of California in 1973, taking on a scholar-in-residence position at a place called the Esalen Institute.

Grof's work in the 1970s was profoundly influential to a collective of young psychonauts. His philosophy for LSD therapy involved what he at the time called one's 'inner radar'. Trying to build a philosophical foundation for how psychedelic medicine worked, Grof first described his ideas this way:

> This specific affinity of LSD for emotionally highly charged dynamic structures has significant diagnostic

> and therapeutic implications. Because of this unusual property, LSD can be used as a kind of 'inner radar' that scans the unconscious, identifies the areas of high affective tension, and brings them to the open. It helps the patient and the therapist to distinguish relevant material from the trivial and unimportant, establish proper hierarchies of priorities, and recognise the most urgent areas for therapeutic work.[35]

As Grof's ideas evolved at Esalen, MDMA emerged to light a fire under all the old psychedelic therapists who had been stifled by governmental controls on psychedelics in the 1960s. MDMA seemed to be a perfect therapy drug, doing all the things LSD did but with fewer negative side effects. MDMA was shorter acting than LSD. It more reliably promoted positive moods. It didn't 'threaten ego control' like LSD, and was simply much easier to direct therapeutically.[36]

By that point Grof had developed his ideas to the point that they transcended LSD specifically and were more about the way entering 'non-ordinary states of consciousness' could be a universal tool for potentiating all kinds of healing. Drugs, of course, were the simplest and most effective way to enter those states, but Grof also broadly accepted everything from hypnosis to breathwork to meditation as useful triggers. According to Grof's thesis, once we are inside those transitory phenomenological spaces, our bodies naturally excavate troubling material. 'Entering these states activates an inner self-healing intelligence, which automatically guides the process to unconscious material that has a strong emotional charge and is close to the threshold of consciousness,' Grof wrote. 'It then spontaneously brings this material to the surface for processing.'[37]

Reading Grof's work quickly draws you into some strange places. As Grof went deeper into the idea that buried trauma underpins most psychosomatic disorders, his work ended up at what he believed to be the first, and biggest, trauma we all experience: birth.

Grof believes we all carry a trauma memory of our birth. This memory is powerful and lucid, and it has fundamental ramifications for our emotional and psychological resilience as adults. Using MDMA to relive our birth memory is one crucial way Grof believes the drug aids healing.

The MAPS manual somewhat cleverly dilutes Grof's original idea by avoiding the striking phrase 'birth trauma' and replacing it with a more semantically gentle note suggesting that therapists should be aware of 'perinatal and/or spiritual experiences' emerging during the drug sessions. The training manual also makes clear that therapists must not challenge the veracity of these emergent experiences because this is just the body's inner healing intelligence doing the beneficial work.[38]

Eventually Grof's ideas went even further back in time, before one's birth. His views ultimately landed in the world of past-life experiences, and his descriptions of how to manage these 'past-life memories' are clear.[39] It's important to stress that Grof is not talking in metaphor here. He genuinely believes the past-life memories that materialise during a drug experience are real:

> On a deeper level, the symptoms [of mental health problems] are related to the trauma of birth and even to physical traumas associated with past-life memories. The material underlying psychosomatic pains can include memories of accidents, operations, or diseases from infancy, childhood, and later life, the pain experienced during the birth process, and physical suffering connected with injuries or death in a previous incarnation.[40]

While the MAPS manual for MDMA therapy is careful to avoid referencing some of Grof's more out-there beliefs, the head of MAPS and driver of much of today's modern psychedelic renaissance, Rick Doblin, often professes his admiration for Grof. In 2015, Doblin explicitly made clear the 'entire therapeutic approach we have in the MDMA studies' is based on the teachings of Stan Grof. Doblin explained the essence of the inner-healing mechanism in MDMA work is due to Grof's 'death–rebirth process'.[41]

WHEN AUSTRALIA'S TGA MADE ITS MOMENTOUSLY unexpected decision in 2023 to reschedule MDMA and psilocybin, it did so with a peculiar lack of detail. Being only a drug regulator, the TGA recognised it had no way to control how clinicians were ultimately going to use these drugs in practice. What kind of therapeutic container should accompany use of these drugs? That wasn't a question for the TGA to answer. It wasn't a question the TGA *could* answer.

Instead, the government body could only 'recommend' clinicians look to 'guidelines' from professional organisations such as the Royal Australian and New Zealand College of Psychiatrists (RANZCP).

The RANZCP has conspicuously avoided directly recommending any one of the several psychedelic therapist training programs emerging in Australia. It did, however, publish a 'training framework'. The brief three-page document, first published in 2023, offered a vague dot-pointed checklist for psychiatrists to use when evaluating the standard of any given training course in Australia. At the end of the document, three resources were listed as suggested therapy methodologies for psychedelic work. One of those references was the MAPS training manual.[42]

An update to the document was published in June 2025. The only edit to the original version was to make crystal clear that 'the RANZCP does not endorse any individual training program'.

'I'M AN MDMA RESEARCHER, NOT A PSYCHEDELIC RESEARCHER'

This MAPS model isn't the only way MDMA therapy is being practised in Australia, but it certainly is the primary way it is being practised in the real world. Because the TGA authorised MDMA for treating PTSD, and because this paradigm was the most advanced in clinical trials, it is unsurprising to find that the 'inner healer excavating repressed trauma memories' model is so dominant in Australian therapeutic circles.

I wanted to find some people doing it differently. And to find them I had to jump back into the world of clinical trials and academia.

Gillinder Bedi is not a psychedelic researcher. 'I'm an MDMA researcher,' she emphatically tells me. And running through her bio quickly affirms that while she certainly doesn't have much of a background working with classic psychedelics, she likely is one of the most experienced MDMA researchers in Australia today.

Bedi's early years were spent at Monash University training in clinical psychology, with a 2006 PhD focusing on how recreational ecstasy use affects memory. Completing her PhD, she moved to the United States to continue investigating the effects of MDMA in humans. After all, as we've seen, if you were interested in working with drugs like MDMA in Australia in the late 2000s and early 2010s, you would be basically banging your head against a brick wall.

First at the University of Chicago, and then at Columbia University Irving Medical Center in New York City, Bedi spent nearly ten years working with MDMA in the US. Decades of anecdotal study into recreational uses of ecstasy had been clear about why people seemed to enjoy taking this drug – its profound prosocial effects, the way users felt more deeply connected to others – but Bedi's studies offered some of the first real clinical investigations into the way MDMA alters people's social experiences.

By 2017, Bedi got back to Australia and joined an organisation called Orygen. Founded in the 1980s as a small research unit focused on youth mental health, Orygen had slowly grown in prominence until, in 2018, it opened a massive translational research institute in Parkville, Melbourne. Here, Bedi started to pull all her interests together as she explored some novel ways to utilise MDMA as an adjunct to psychotherapy.

Looking at the MAPS model of MDMA therapy for PTSD left Bedi confused. Why would you take a drug like MDMA and use it to direct a person to focus on internal feelings? It didn't make sense to her. 'It seemed to me that [the MAPS model] wasn't really utilising the main sort of bang for your buck you get with MDMA, which is the social effects,' Bedi observed. 'That's one of the key features that differentiate this medication from classic psychedelics.'

Also, as a clinical psychologist, Bedi was baffled by the way the MAPS model presented the idea of the inner healer. It was strange to consider MDMA as some kind of special medicine where you put on an eye mask and let it show you what you need to learn. That certainly wasn't what she knew MDMA to be, after years of researching it.

So what *could* MDMA be really useful for?

Bedi began working with Adam Guastella, a neurodiversity expert and professor from the University of Sydney. Guastella had developed a therapeutic program to help manage social anxiety in young people with autism, and Bedi's knowledge of

MDMA's prosocial effects led them to wonder whether the two modalities could be combined to create a novel treatment.

To Bedi it felt like a perfect match of drug and disorder – and so emerged a unique clinical trial dubbed PAPAYA (Pharmacologically-Assisted Psychotherapy for Social Anxiety in Young People with Autism).

Aiming to run until late 2027, the trial focuses on young adults (aged 16 to 25) with a relatively recent diagnosis of autism and a clinical diagnosis of social anxiety disorder. The trial is placebo-controlled, with three separate active placebo groups to be compared with the MDMA cohort.

The most exciting part of Bedi's trial design is the novelty of the dose sessions. There is no lying down quietly with eye masks and headphones here. Instead, the researchers want to use the time participants are under the influence of MDMA to do active therapy work.

One exercise the participants will engage in is called imagery rescripting. This is a common psychotherapy technique in which a patient accesses a memory that is linked to a specific negative feeling. That memory is approached then with an alternative perspective, allowing a new positive experience to essentially rewrite the negative sense. Could MDMA amplify the effectiveness of this therapeutic process?

Another exercise planned for the dose sessions is a kind of formal exposure therapy. In the case of someone with social anxiety, the exposure would be communicating with a stranger. Here, the researchers plan to have a member of the team who is a stranger to the participant enter the room at a time when the MDMA is working and have a conversation. 'We view the MDMA sessions as almost a type of behavioural experiment, and what's changing is not the experience per se, but the way people feel when they're having those experiences because of the medication,' Bedi explains.

The way Bedi's team is approaching MDMA therapy in their trial is wildly different to anything in current clinical use. There are still the usual preparation and integration therapy sessions on either side of the dose day, but when the participants are under the influence of the drug they will be actively doing therapeutic work.

IT DOESN'T TAKE LONG TALKING TO BEDI BEFORE THE elephant in the room again emerges: the Bessel van der Kolk of it all.

Once pushed to the sidelines of credibility as a 'casualty of the memory wars',[43] van der Kolk has now returned to the mainstream, propped up on the wave of psychedelic medicine. His now iconic, bestselling book *The Body Keeps the Score* was only a minor success when it was published in 2014, but it reached new heights from 2021 onwards, and by late 2025 it had surpassed three million in sales.

In his book, MDMA barely gets more than a page or two of discussion, and van der Kolk's description of the drug is strikingly uninformed.[44] At some point, however, his ideas about trauma intermingled with the MAPS framework of MDMA therapy. They were a match made in heaven: van der Kolk's work presented a pop-science foundation for trauma that MDMA seemed perfectly poised to fix. Today, he is deeply intertwined in the world of MDMA therapy. He is co-author on several journal articles reporting late-stage MAPS clinical trial results, and frequently appears as a guest lecturer in psychedelic therapy training programs.

Gill Bedi has worked long enough in the field of substance-abuse problems to know how profound childhood trauma can be for many patients. But the idea that 'everything is trauma' rang as absurd. To her it's worryingly simplistic to suggest we just need to address some buried trauma and then all our other problems will just go away. 'I just think it's very reductive. Obviously, it's a great name for a book: *The Body Keeps the Score*. It's incredibly intuitive. People really buy into it.'

But, asks Bedi, why are we not focusing on using MDMA therapeutically for the things that the drug seems to do best?

Years of research showed Bedi that MDMA was a wildly prosocial drug. Its unique magic is in the way it weakens a person's sense of separation from others. Those invisible barriers that make us feel alone, different and disconnected all fade away under the influence of MDMA. Of course, this is also why it's a perfect party drug. Hundreds of people aren't exactly going to raves and collectively unearthing childhood trauma memories together.

No. They are sharing in a moment of connection. So if we were to utilise this feeling therapeutically, we'd want to work on the way the drug affects our external interactions with others.

At the end of our conversation Bedi dropped one incredible idea in the mix that felt a little like a grenade left in one's wake. Her next clinical trial aim is looking at MDMA interventions in people with antisocial personality traits.

'What do you mean?' I asked. 'Like people with narcissism?'

'Oh, not just that,' Bedi replied. She was talking about participants with empathy problems, going all the way to those with criminally aggressive behaviour. How is it we have a drug we know generates prosocial feelings of empathy, and we are not using it to help people who have difficulties with empathy?

Could MDMA therapy be a way to help rehabilitate those with antisocial traits? And how early in a person's life should it be utilised? If antisocial behaviour is one of the leading pathways into substance-use disorders in young people, what if we could help those young people regain a sense of empathy and connectedness?

After talking to Bedi, I was left with a whole host of new

questions. I mean, giving drugs to rehabilitate criminals is undoubtedly a slippery slope into *A Clockwork Orange* territory. And how young is too young if we're thinking about giving children mind-altering drugs to modify their behaviour? We already do it with stimulants and ADHD, I guess. But where's the line here? Is there even a line?

Aside from a mind spinning with novel thoughts, perhaps the biggest lingering question I had about modern MDMA-assisted therapy was: how did we get here? How did some pretty unusual New Age ideas get so intertwined with MDMA therapy, and become so entrenched that they became the primary operating system for a whole new wave of clinical medicine?

I needed to come out and say the big question I was really skirting around. How did psychedelic medicine become such a magnet for pseudoscientific woo?

THE REVOLUTION HAS BEEN INTERNALISED

Repressed memories, inner healing intelligence, holotropic breathwork, EMDR, meditation, past-life regression, birth trauma. When entering the world of psychedelic medicine, it doesn't take long before you are dealing with ideas that blur the line between science and spirituality. I've been reporting on psychedelic science and medicine for nearly a decade and I've seen rooms where drug-dosing sessions are conducted. Most carry some sign of what we would call a New Age belief.

Inside the famous psilocybin dosing rooms at Johns Hopkins University in the early 2000s sat statues of Buddha and prehistoric mushroom figurines. Other rooms I have seen carry Tibetan singing bowls, salt crystal lamps, sticks of sage to burn, quartz crystals, and even intention cards with motivational aphorisms.

One of Australia's biggest psychedelic therapist training

programs – spanning 12 months, 200 hours and a $7000 fee – claims to be 'rooted in the contemplative traditions of Yoga and Buddhism'.[45] Electives for the course at time of writing included breathwork, Vedic meditation and music yoga therapy. The course also includes clinical placements, giving participants direct experience supervising real-world psychedelic therapy dosing sessions. And it's a registered training course, counting as professional development for Australia's peak representative bodies for psychiatrists and psychologists.

The integration of modern psychedelic medicine with New Age spiritual beliefs is virtually impossible to avoid. There is no way someone who wants to get involved with using these drugs clinically can escape this wholesale amalgam of New Age spiritual woo and hard psychedelic science.

But how did we get here?

WHEN PSYCHEDELICS SLIPPED OUT OF CLINICS AND labs in the 1960s, they landed into a culture undergoing a massive transformation. In the United States there was a revolution brewing. Protests were everywhere. Protests against war, government, corporate consumerism. People fighting for civil rights, human rights. In this blistering environment, psychedelics served as a kind of revolutionary rocket fuel. Taking LSD became an act of political defiance. The drug bonded, and boosted, powerful activist groups, from the Black Panthers to the Weather Underground's militant Marxists.

In Adam Curtis's monumental documentary series *The Century of the Self*, the underlying philosophy of the youth protest movement in the late 1960s is summed up by a slogan coined by controversial philosopher Herbert Marcuse: 'There is a policeman inside all our heads. He must be destroyed.'

The idea, Marcuse surmised, was that capitalist systems of

control, perpetuated by corporations and the state, were keeping people brainwashed and idle. Violent destruction of these systems was the only way to liberate the people.

'We want to live a life that isn't based on materialistic values and yet the whole system of government and the economy of America is based on profit; on personal greed and selfishness so that in order to be human, in order to love each other, and be equal with each other, and not place each other in roles, we have to destroy the kind of government that keeps us from asserting our positive values of life,'[46] explained Linda Evans, a member of the Weather Underground, in the documentary.

But as Curtis deftly explained, the state fought back with violent force. Protests were quashed, students were killed, and government agencies like the FBI relentlessly hunted down revolutionary groups, labelling them terrorists. So how could one liberate oneself from the tyranny of society and overcome the policeman inside our heads?

'People who had been politically active were persuaded that if they could change themselves and be healthy individuals, and if a movement grew up just aimed at people changing themselves, then at some point, with all that positive change going on ... there would be a sort of a spontaneous transformation of society,' explained activist Stew Albert.[47]

This retreat into the self became a powerful directive force for the counterculture in the 1970s. After being completely suppressed by the state, the rebellion turned inward. If you change your mind, then the world will follow. The revolution will not be televised; it had been internalised.

And there was a group in California ready to take up the philosophical mantle for all these psychedelic refugees.

The group was called the Esalen Institute, and across the 1960s it slowly became influential in the counterculture movement. Esalen was the home of a philosophy that eventually became known as the human potential movement, which spun out of an idea from American psychologist Abraham Maslow dubbed the hierarchy of human needs. Maslow's hierarchy became a kind of blueprint for those chasing self-betterment.

There were five steps to Maslow's hierarchy, and as a person moved through each stage – physiological, safety, belonging and love, esteem and self-actualisation needs – they got closer to a state of supreme self-transcendence. This was the realisation of one's true potential and in this moment of ultimate insight one would transcend all of society's imprisoning constructs.

Esalen's goal was to map out a path to help people reach their true potential. By the early 1970s, it had completely captured the counterculture zeitgeist. Political activism was over. The left-leaning student protests had failed. The revolution was now all about freeing one's mind. The psychedelic world had become fixated with healing 'the self', and from here we saw the birth of the New Age movement.

A group called the Association for the Responsible Use of Psychedelic Agents (ARUPA) was formed at Esalen in 1978. Its goal was to informally steer the direction of therapeutic uses of psychedelics. By the early 1980s, MDMA was the topic du jour. Everyone had seen how things had deteriorated with psychedelic medicines in the 1960s and were consciously working to keep MDMA from suffering the same fate.

Invitation lists at ARUPA meetings were like a who's who of psychedelic culture: Leo Zeff, Ralph Metzner, Stan Grof, Rick Strassman, a young Rick Doblin. Everything around MDMA and Esalen coalesced during an invite-only conference convened by ARUPA in March 1985.[48] Thirty-five people were at the meeting and it was clear the days were numbered for legal MDMA uses. The US government was working hard to move MDMA through the hoops necessary to make it a Schedule 1 drug. Halfway through the five-day ARUPA meeting, around a third of the participants took part in an 'experiential session', taking MDMA with a therapist.

Spoiler alert: ARUPA failed in its quest to stifle the scheduling of MDMA. By mid-1985 the drug had been hit with an emergency scheduling order by the DEA. Within a year it was formally scheduled. MDMA was illegal, and Rick Doblin began a new multi-decade project to make the drug available again to therapists.

It's crucial to understand that nearly everyone currently driving psychedelic medicine today can in some way, either literally or philosophically, be drawn back to the ebbs and flows of work at Esalen in the 1970s and '80s. Stan Grof is cited as a deep influence on a massive swathe of contemporary psychedelic scientists. Esalen also paved the way for the influx of New Age gurus in the late 20th century. Gabor Maté, Rupert Sheldrake, Deepak Chopra: all at some point engaged with Esalen, and all, in the 21st century, became guiding forces in the psychedelic medicine movement.

What we end up with is psychedelics in the age of 'me'. An era of the self, culminating in a drive for drugs to help us heal the self. As Peter Marin succinctly described in his prescient 1975 essay 'The New Narcissism', Western culture had swerved from being simply individualistic to something more akin to narcissism.[49] Our obsessions in the 1980s and '90s with self-help, self-improvement, psychotherapy and general New Age spiritualism all fed into a culture of capitalism. Do this course, buy this book. Become the most authentic version of you. Find your true self.

Maslow's ideal of self-actualisation had become Western culture's perfect commodity. And with psychedelic medicine thrown into the mix, a new tool was commodified for inner exploration. A tool that helps us explore our own inner world. A tool that helps us find our truest self.

Step right up, step right up, step right up: Ancient Plant Medicine™ is all you need to become the best version of you.

Psychedelic science in the 2020s has pursued this monomaniacal focus on the self into a strange medicalised space. We relentlessly push classic psychedelics into the container of medicines but forget to engage with the potential novelty of these substances. I myself have had experiences with both psychedelics and our modern mental healthcare system. And after all this investigating, I still struggle to understand how the two things effectively intertwine. I can't help but wonder: are we doing this all wrong?

6
FUTURES

WHAT IF WE'RE DOING IT ALL WRONG?

'Drugs, which can be helpful when wisely used, become dangerous when foolishly used. The sudden insight becomes "all," and the patient and disciplined "working through" is postponed or devalued. Instead of being "surprised by joy," "turning on" is scheduled, promised, advertised, sold, hustled into being, and can get to be regarded as a commodity.'

Abraham Maslow, *Religions, Values, and Peak-Experiences*, Penguin, 1976 (original work 1964), p. x

It all started with a jittery leg.

I'd sit on the sofa every evening and my leg would quietly bounce up and down. Initially it almost felt like a conscious affectation. I knew I was doing it but there wasn't a problem. After all, we were in the first months of the Covid pandemic in 2020; everyone was stuck at home and a little bit of stewing anxiety was to be expected.

The rest of the year was rough. Against a background of rolling lockdowns, my partner faced two miscarriages, my father died and I suffered from kidney stones. If any year was going to proffer a hit to my mental health, it was going to be 2020.

But life went on, the knots of anxiety normalised, and a few objectively wonderful things happened. A healthy pregnancy emerged and a beautiful girl was born in 2022. I persevered, playing the role of stoic partner and new dad. But things were getting harder. I wasn't happy. Parenthood amplified the social isolation seeded by the pandemic, and then I stopped working in 2023 to take over the reins of primary parent.

Here, things started getting impossible to ignore. My moods were erratic. I was exhausted all the time. Things were just ... inexplicably sad. Butting up against those feelings were all the proclamations from people on the outside telling me how special this time was. What a privilege. Except it didn't *feel* that way.

So, what do you do when experiencing a mental health crisis in 21st-century Australia? Well, first you try to fix it yourself. Exercise more. See friends. You know what you need to do to make yourself feel better. Every intervention was obvious and I'd engage for a week or two before slipping back into inactive doldrums.

After a few months it became clear I needed some kind of specialist help. First step: visit my GP. I like my local GP, and I don't disparage any of his methods or advice. He talked me through a mental health plan. Recommended a local psychologist and started me on a generic SSRI antidepressant. Pretty routine stuff. Come back in a month or so and we'll review the dose, he suggested. Okey dokey.

A month later, when I was still feeling flat, we upped the antidepressant dose. I also started seeing the psychologist I'd been referred to: a young psychology graduate in her thirties, and perfectly procedural in her consultations.

More time passed; the waves of fatigue increased. And then side effects from the antidepressant started hitting me hard. I was sleeping more than I should have been. I felt flat, or 'emotionally blunted', as the textbooks like to say. My GP did the right thing and switched me to a different drug. Let's try something else. Okey dokey.

Three sessions into the psychology work and things were progressing as blandly as one would expect. We had a 'breakthrough'. The psychologist 'discovered' some medical disruptions in my teenage years that were of course the source of all my problems. Childhood trauma – ding, ding, ding. This was a surprise to no one other than the psychologist.

The new antidepressant medication certainly fixed my fatigue problem. I wasn't as tired as with the other drug. Now I was just hyper-jittery and anxious. I felt like a pinball being bounced around a machine. Another month or two passed, another GP visit, another increase to my drug dose. Apparently the anxiety would decrease as my body got used to the drug. Okey dokey.

I stopped seeing the psychologist. We weren't clicking. And the new antidepressant was making me feel more erratic and unstable than ever. It had been about nine months since I'd started on this journey through mental health treatment and, to be honest, I think I was worse than when I'd started. The drugs had made me feel more destabilised, chipping away at what little psychological resilience I had left. I was getting viscerally upset at small things; I yelled at local coffee shop workers for taking too long to make my coffee.

By mid-2024 things had completely fallen apart. I was in tears almost every other day, entirely dysfunctional and barely able to take care of myself, let alone my partner and daughter.

I ended up being admitted as an inpatient to a nearby psychiatric hospital, about to get a firsthand insight into modern mental healthcare and the often erratic way that psychiatric medicines are prescribed.

MEDICINES AND DRUGS

For most of this book I have, perhaps flippantly, used the words 'medicine' and 'drug' in interchangeable ways. Of course not all medicines are drugs, and not all drugs are medicines. Our binary frameworks tend to perceive medicines as good and drugs as bad. I know that it's easy to pull that idea apart (I'm looking at you, caffeine and alcohol) but in terms of the way value judgments are apportioned to uses of substances, it's certainly socially preferable to call something a medicine over a drug. Consider yourself not a psychedelic *drug* user but a psychedelic *medicine* user.

So how, then, do we make whole the idea of psychedelics if these substances are both drugs (bad) *and* medicines (good)?

We need to grapple with semantics for a second, and I promise I won't fall into the triteness of writing something like, 'As defined by the *Oxford English Dictionary*, a medicine is …' Nevertheless, we do need to consider what exactly the word 'medicine' means when we consider it in the context of the phrase 'psychedelic medicine'.

In the province of Western thought, we generally operate in a binary between sick and well. When you're sick, you visit a doctor. The doctor diagnoses the illness and prescribes medicine to cure or relieve your symptoms.

Thus, the process of *medicalising* psychedelics is one by which scientists work to understand what diseases these drugs can treat, and establish processes by which clinicians can use those drugs as medicines to make people better.

Although there are plenty of exceptions (again, I'll never forget you, caffeine and alcohol), in modern Western societies we generally don't look kindly on *drug use* when it's taken outside of a formal medical container. Drug use that isn't explicitly considered medicinal is framed as 'recreational', and considered poor behaviour. Outside of the socially allowed 'vices' (which are not considered 'drugs' in the conventional sense), we shun drug use that isn't prescribed to a patient by a clinician.

In fact, once a drug has been explicitly categorised as a medicine, its uses outside of that medical container become especially illicit, loaded with socially or morally punitive outcomes. Psilocybin, for example, may now be acceptable as a medicine for treatment-resistant depression, but if you take magic mushrooms in any other context, even with an intent to heal, you are fundamentally engaging in drug abuse.

As anthropologist Tehseen Noorani puts it, 'In providing frameworks for "proper use," medicalisation delineates the conditions of "abuse."'[1] Noorani suggests most modern psychedelic clinical trials are so narrowly focused on specific doses and diseases they contribute to the ongoing idea that any uses beyond this frame are illicit.

In a conscious strategy designed to dismantle the 'drug' container psychedelics have been dropped into over the past 70 years, there is a popular aphorism commonly used by those advocating or evangelising psychedelic use. In fact, I'm sure you have heard it. It opens many a news article or even science article talking about psychedelics.[2]

You see: psychedelics have been used for thousands of years by cultures all around the world for healing. These are *natural plant medicines,* not *drugs.*

The messaging is relentless and it's powerful. It's a statement so often repeated that it is now just taken for granted. It is never questioned. But is it true?

COMMON, ANCIENT, MEDICINE

Manvir Singh, a professor of anthropology at the University of California at Davis, has been investigating this question for nearly 15 years. Alongside long fieldwork stints in Indonesia, Vanuatu and Colombia, Singh fully catalysed his ideas into a book, published in 2025, titled *Shamanism: The Timeless Religion.*[3]

In the book Singh presented what he calls the Global Archaic Psychedelic Shamanism hypothesis, reduced to an amusing acronym: GAPS. According to Singh there are three claims we are working with:

Psychedelic use has been widespread across the world.

Psychedelic use is ancient, going back thousands of years.

Psychedelics were used by shamans, or cultural equivalents of healers, for therapeutic purposes.

So how true are those three claims?

We can approach the first two claims together. Have people all over the world been using psychedelics for thousands of years?

Rather surprisingly, Singh's conclusion is, 'Probably not.' There is actually very little evidence this is true, and to come close to validating that statement people often quickly broaden the terms they are using.

References to classic psychedelics, as we have established to be those chemicals that stimulate 5-HT2A receptors, are surprisingly rare in both anthropological and mythological literature. One of Singh's investigations led him to scan a massive resource called the eHRAF. Housed at Yale University, this is a collection of almost 7000 books and articles investigating 325 different cultural groups around the world.

Singh looked at how often these texts contained references to different natural psychoactive substances. Mushrooms barely made an entrance into the list, coming up in just 22 different paragraphs across 19 cultures. And looking with a granular eye into those references, the vast majority were simply of mushrooms as background scenery in stories.

Peyote (mescaline) was perhaps the most referenced classic psychedelic in his investigations, with 308 mentions. However, these mentions only spanned ten different cultures, solely situated in the region of Central America.

These findings of psychedelic use can be contrasted with the incredibly broad amount of references to more popular, less medicinally used intoxicants, including 166 mentions of beer across 43 cultures, and 465 mentions of tobacco across 85 cultures.

Turns out psychedelic use may not be that common around the world, but we certainly love a smoke and a drink.

On the 'ancient' side of the fence, Singh raised some strikingly provocative ideas about how recent psychedelic use may be in some indigenous cultures. Investigating ayahuasca, for example, led him to conclude this well-known ritual brew possibly diffused across the Amazon as recently as over the last 300 years. Ayahuasca use may be ancient, but Singh speculates these older uses were possibly not widespread, likely restricted to a small, localised region.

These ideas are inarguably controversial. The ayahuasca origins debate is a hot one in psychedelic anthropological circles. But more generally, these debates challenge many modern psychedelic advocates in their belief of how traditional these drugs have been.

For me, however, the most confronting – and convincing – part of Singh's argument comes when we dig into the third oft-heard claim: that psychedelics were used by shamans as medicines for therapeutic healing.

The common characterisation of traditional shamanic healing is that psychedelics were historically only administered for clear, circumscribed reasons to individuals with severe medical or psychological problems.[4] Singh sees this as a fundamentally misleading way to frame traditional uses of psychedelics.

Perhaps the biggest fallacy in the traditional psychedelic medicine paradigm is the idea that people who need healing are given a psychedelic substance. Singh suggests it can be rare in traditional contexts for a regular person to consume a psychedelic brew. In many cases, where someone presents to a local shaman with a psychological or physical illness, the shaman would often be the one to take the psychedelic. They would enter a spirit realm and cleanse the person of whatever demonic energy was responsible for their ailment.

As an example, Singh cites an infamous documentary from the 1970s that chronicles the ceremonial rituals of a group known as the Yanomami in Venezuela. In the film we see shamans in the group consume a powerful snuff we now know contains DMT. This ceremony is performed to serve a number of purposes, from cleansing the village of evil spirits to sending those evil spirits to attack a nearby village. As the shamans fall under the thrall of the drug, they begin to role-play a violent scenario in which babies in the neighbouring village are murdered. As Singh explains:

> Anthropological research conducted since the mid-twentieth century shows that, among the Yanomami and many other groups, shamans use psychedelics to tap into the supernatural and provide services like weather change, divination, physical healing, and aggressive

> sorcery. They might confront heinous sorcerers. They might purge patients of treacherous ghosts. They might become supernatural beings themselves. Psychedelics – like dancing, drumming, darkness, and other psychotropic drugs – push shamans into a state where they and their communities believe them to access otherworldly powers. This contrasts with the Western clinical application, where psychedelics are administered like medicine and used to break down patients' harmful patterns of thought.[5]

Singh goes on to discuss how modern uses of psychedelics in traditional South American contexts have been deeply shaped by European colonialism. Current modes of ayahuasca tourism, for example, where Westerners travel to parts of the Amazon and take 'the medicine', are often performative experiences designed to pander to our ideas of a traditional indigenous ceremony. According to Singh, the way shamanic healers deliver psychedelics to Western tourists often diverges dramatically from how they would do things normally among their own people.

Ultimately, this vision of psychedelics as *ancient healing medicine* is a powerfully narrow perspective, and one that is often propagated as a way of challenging Western taboos. Even more worrying, this view oversimplifies and removes specificity from traditional cultural uses.

This isn't to suggest psychedelics aren't helpful to many people, especially within the ceremonial modalities that we are talking about. I don't think there is anything wrong with someone travelling to Peru to take ayahuasca as part of a self-healing journey. There is no doubt that psychedelics can be profound healing tools for some people. But it does seem important to not whitewash or misconstrue ancient traditions as a way of making ourselves feel better about how we choose to utilise psychedelic drugs in the 21st century.

Ancient psychedelic uses were likely extraordinarily diverse, philosophically complicated and quite unlike what we are doing today in modern medicine. We have taken something that was possibly used by a small number of indigenous cultures and rewritten their stories to fit our biases. In some ways, one could argue that we are flattening, or even erasing, those diverse indigenous stories by marginalising ancient psychedelic use into our simplistic modern framework of 'medicine'.

IS THIS REALLY HOW WE DO IT?

As someone steeped in popular culture, my touchstones for psychiatric hospital were from movies. Was I about to befriend a wild kindred spirit whose energy would offer me a new perspective on life? Or would I battle a stern matron who was treating all the patients poorly? Maybe I'd be just passingly amused by the paranoid rantings of a schizophrenic questioning reality?

Turns out it was nothing like any of that. My time in psychiatric hospital was banal, boring and uneventful.

After a check-in process that involved my bags being searched for things with which I could harm myself, I was left alone in a barren room to spend my days binge-watching streaming television. On the first day my assigned psychiatrist came by to visit and explain the looming process. I wasn't in hospital to explore my mind in group therapy sessions, but instead the time was primarily being used to stabilise my mental state using drugs. Lots of drugs. (Or should I say 'medicines'?)

My time in hospital would be best used, I was told, to swiftly titrate different drug doses. By being observed so closely, I could rapidly move up and down drug doses while the doctors worked out what was best for me. The first step would be giving me drugs/medicine to sleep, alongside a switch back to an antidepressant

I'd previously been on, 'just so we can understand how you respond'.

You can probably guess how I was a few days later: a jittery, doped-up cliché of the drugged-out psychiatric patient. More days passed – a little less of one drug and a little more of another. It felt like I was a lab rat, with researchers throwing random things at me to see what would happen.

When I made this observation months later to a different psychiatrist, he openly, and sadly, responded with, 'Yeah, that is pretty much the way we do it.' I couldn't believe how scattershot modern mental health medicine was. Part of me assumed our medical knowledge was more precise, more knowing.

But nope. We don't even know how lots of these drugs actually work, and we have no way to know exactly what is going to work for a given patient. The treatment protocol is literally: 'Try some of this. How do you feel? Worse? Okay, try some of this, then.' I think my description of the process at the time was, 'So it's like throwing shit at the wall and seeing what sticks?'

After a couple of weeks, we ended up with a conventional SSRI antidepressant and I was sent home. The bracing experience of being admitted into a psychiatric hospital acted a little like a circuit breaker. It was humbling, it was isolating, and I guess it served as a kind of rock bottom. Over the next few months, I would work with a therapist and try to find a way forward.

By the end of 2024, I was better, at least relatively. The right drugs at the right time were helpful. I can confidently say that. However, the entire, multi-year process of moving through our modern mental healthcare system left me feeling broken.

I had so many questions. Is this really how we do things? Is this the best way to help people suffering mental health crises? And, perhaps most pertinently, as I'd been reporting on psychedelic medicine for so many years: how the hell were we going to integrate psychedelic drugs into this system?

While in hospital I considered what it would be like to be in a world where patients in these environments were given psychedelic drugs. Maybe just down the hall was a treatment room where we'd go and spend a few hours having a dose of something. Truly, the thought at the time horrified me. Not only was this space about as far from the kind of optimal set and setting I'd be comfortable 'tripping' in, but the mental image of a room where you would be given 'the medicine' felt almost dystopian. Go in upset and defeated; come out a few hours later happy, light, joyous. In the context of our current psychiatric hospital system, it seemed like *Manchurian Candidate* levels of brainwashing.

Closing in on the definition of 'treatment-resistant', I now technically qualify for psychedelic medicine in Australia, at least within the strict diagnostic framework we currently use. But it seemed crazy to me that I needed to get this sick, this destabilised, before I was 'fit' for psychedelic medicine. The whole thing felt back to front. Why are we waiting until people reach rock bottom before we give them powerful mind-altering drugs that may, or may not, help them? After all I'd been through, I wondered whether psilocybin or MDMA would be the best thing for me now. Was I harder to treat after going through such a rigmarole?

What would have happened if I'd had the option of getting these drugs a few years earlier? Before things got really bad. I mean, I'm not psychedelically naive. I know what these drugs are like. The thought of taking any psychedelic drug in the moments I was most unstable felt absolutely frightening.

One massive question bounced around my mind. Are we doing psychedelic medicine all wrong?

THE MODERN PSYCHEDELIC CLINIC

When the TGA in Australia made the unexpected decision to allow MDMA and psilocybin for limited medical uses in 2023, a number of clinicians and corporations jumped into action. For many, the 'psychedelic '20s' were kicking into gear. Rick Doblin had been travelling the globe for years delivering inspirational utopian lectures describing a future where psychedelic clinics were on every other street corner. Mental healthcare would be transformed.

Phase 1 of this grand plan was the kind of regulatory approval Australia had enacted. And what should quickly follow was the emergence of thousands and thousands of psychedelic clinics delivering MDMA, psilocybin, ketamine, and whatever other psychedelic drugs that were coming down the line. As new drugs were approved for more conditions, the clinics could become your one-stop mental healthcare shop.

By early 2024, Australia's first dedicated, purpose-built psychedelic clinic had opened. Situated on the edge of the Yarra River in Melbourne's leafy inner-city suburbs, Clarion Clinics' name said it all. This was a call to action. A notice to everyone, not only in Australia but the world, that the psychedelic clinic revolution had begun.

Less than 12 months after Clarion Clinics opened its doors with a flurry of hyperbolic press releases, it closed them ever so quietly. By mid-2025, the clinic was a distant memory, only traceable using the internet's time machine. The location had been taken over by another organisation keen to give psychedelic medicine a shot, but the original Clarion founders had retreated.

Why did Australia's first psychedelic clinic shut its doors so quickly?

Was it too soon? Maybe.

Was it too expensive? Definitely.

After switching on in 2023, pretty much everyone in Australia quickly realised psychedelic medicine was not going to be easy to roll out or scale up. The paradigm authorised by the country's regulator gestured to the protocols used in recent clinical trials. Running someone through a course of psychedelic medicine would take at least three months, often longer. That time would involve around a dozen psychotherapy sessions, including longer preparatory visits with a prescribing psychiatrist. And dose days were even more labour intensive.

Modern clinical practice generally has psychedelic doses delivered by a dyad of medical professionals. Two trained clinicians are required to sit with a patient for around eight hours while he or she has their experience. That's 16 hours of medical professional time, per dose. And a treatment course usually includes two to three doses of whatever drug is being used. In Australia, you'd be hard pressed to find a standard psychologist charging less than $200 an hour, let alone a clinical psychologist or a psychiatrist.

Maybe you've jumped ahead of me and done the maths, but psychedelic medicine was proving not cheap. The first wave of psychedelic therapy practitioners in Australia were charging anywhere from $20 000 to $35 000 for a treatment course. Even the more creative clinicians I have spoken to, who worked hard to mitigate costs with Medicare rebates, were still hitting price points around $16 000.

Friends of mine who like playing with numbers spent many a night in 2024 crunching the economics of how a psychedelic clinic could make money. Clarion Clinics, for example, opened with a grand statement of having 'seven treatment rooms' alongside a 'bespoke nine-month psychedelic-assisted therapy program'. Its initial announcement suggested it was a clinic prototype capable of treating around 600 patients per year.

Those kinds of patient numbers are certainly possible, but the human resources necessary to manage so many concurrent dose and therapy sessions quickly becomes head-spinning. A couple of dozen well-trained psychedelic therapists alongside two or three authorised prescriber psychiatrists would be required to keep a clinic chugging along with those numbers. They would all need to be full-time. Just watch your human costs reach millions per year.

Some of the more active voices in the advocacy world suggest the goal right now is to tread water while the first tranche of real-world patients prove these treatments work. From that point, goes the argument, both private and government funding agencies will come on board and suddenly psychedelic clinics will become profitable spaces.

But only thinking about the economics of a dedicated psychedelic clinic can be a red herring. Whether they make financial sense is one thing, but what about considering how these centres would slot into current models of care?

Who, for example, is referring a patient to a psychedelic clinic? If this referral comes from a GP, then what happens to the patient after they receive their quota of allotted psychotherapy? Is that it? No more psychology sessions? Back to your GP?

Or what happens to patients with longstanding relationships with psychologists or psychiatrists? Are they expected to simply port their treatment across to someone else they have no therapeutic alliance with for a few months before returning to their regular clinicians? We know relationships matter in terms of the efficacy of mental health treatments. Is the idea of a treatment model where someone transiently works with a team of therapists for a few months the best way to be doing this?

MORE LIKE A FARMER'S MARKET THAN A WOOLWORTHS

After about a year of working within the conventional clinic-orientated model of psychedelic medicine, Monica Schweickle had a different vision of how this new kind of therapy should be rolled out. Schweickle became frustrated with how expensive and inaccessible the treatment programs were. Being part of the first wave of clinical psychedelic medicine in Australia revealed to her that the model we thought was going to work turned out to be expensive and impractical.

'I think at the beginning everyone was like, "We've got to do exactly what was in the clinical trials. That's what we'll get approved." But now people are realising how individual the treatment needs to be.'

As 2025 progressed Schweickle started up her own business, called The Psychedelic Consultancy. Her goal moved from doing the psychedelic therapy herself with patients to helping psychiatrists get their own authorised prescriber application through the TGA. Instead of patients being shuttled in and out of big psychedelic clinics for apportioned months-long treatments, Schweickle envisions a more functional future in small-scale, community-focused models.

'Psychiatrists who are good psychiatrists want to do this work with their own patients,' Schweickle told me in mid-2025. The more psychiatrists who can be trained up to do the work, the better. The way forward for Schweickle is not, as she puts it, '15 mega clinics across Australia doing the same thing', but an individualised approach with the treatment slotting into more conventional therapy processes. She describes this model as more like a 'farmer's market than a Woolworths'.

Interestingly, the idea Schweickle presented echoed other sentiments that had emerged in conversations I'd had with therapists and clinicians over the course of working on this book.

Coincidently, in late 2025, Paul Liknaitzky and his team at the Monash University Clinical Psychedelic Lab launched a new trial dubbed FIFO-PAT.[6] The acronym for the trial opens out to: a Fly-In Fly-Out model of Psilocybin-Assisted Therapy.

This FIFO model mirrors Schweickle's idea of maintaining treatment continuity between a patient and their regular psychotherapist. Here, the trial will test a scenario whereby a patient's current psychotherapist is paired with a specialist psychedelic therapist. That psychedelic therapist would essentially parachute into a patient's conventional treatment space and accompany the regular therapist on a series of preparatory sessions, culminating in a single drug-dosing day. The psychedelic therapist would then be present for a trio of integration sessions after the dose before 'flying out' of the process to leave the regular psychotherapist and patient to continue with their work.

The FIFO model being tested in the trial spans six weeks and is ostensibly designed to try to find a way to integrate psychedelic medicine into current models of care. It's an exciting way of thinking about psychedelic medicine that eschews the idea of a big, separate psychedelic clinic, and the trial rolls in some fascinating experimental procedures for good measure.

There are three conditions being tested in the trial: the FIFO protocol with reflective journalling, and a treatment-as-usual group serving as control. The third arm, however, introduces a virtual reality component.

Bringing VR into the psychedelic therapy space has long been the vision of researchers Agnieszka Sekula and Prash Puspanathan. Back in 2022, I visited their offices and had a play with some VR software they proposed could be integrated into psychedelic therapy.[7] The general idea is that instead of writing down your insights in a journal following a drug-dosing session, you enter a specifically designed VR environment where thoughts are recorded and visualised as objects like seeds.

The hypothesis is that the VR system can help a patient better access the feelings immediately following a drug session, so that over the next few weeks and months those psychedelic insights can be more effectively integrated into their daily life. In 2022, when I tried the system, it placed me into a beachside environment, where I recorded insights that took the form of floating jewels. Each time I returned to the virtual beach environment, I would revisit those jewel-connected insights and slowly build a three-dimensional map interconnecting those ideas.

It was undeniably a fun, interesting and unusual way of framing a psychotherapy experience, but would it actually help improve therapeutic outcomes? Or was it merely a shiny tech-gimmick? That's still unclear. Adding it as an experimental arm in the FIFO trial will definitely answer some of those questions, and if it does lead to better clinical outcomes, it could be an intriguing new way to reduce the costs of psychedelic medicine.

At the other end of the experimental spectrum in Australia is the idea of inpatient psychedelic clinics. These operate less like an admission to a psychiatric hospital and more like a long-stay rehab centre. In this scenario a patient would spend a stretch of several weeks in a clinic that allows for comprehensive therapy sessions alongside whole-day psychedelic doses.

Before you ask, this mode of psychedelic medicine will not be cheap. This is akin to porting psychedelic medicine into the world of luxury rehab mansions by the beach. One exceptionally exclusive private retreat in Byron Bay has already moved to include a psychedelic-authorised psychiatrist on its staff. In between horseriding, psychotherapy and personal training, you can slot in a few doses of MDMA to really get to that deep trauma at the root of whatever addiction is ailing you. The facility also prides itself on its discretion, suggesting that transport from your destination of choice by private jet can be arranged.

A more grounded, albeit likely still pricey option is a retreat in Melbourne called The Journey Clinic. Calling itself 'the world's first mental-health clinic to specialise in individualised altered-state therapies', this multi-room space in central Melbourne offers bespoke programs individualised to each patient. These programs are framed as three- or four-week residential stays incorporating psychedelic dosing days with a variety of other therapeutic processes.

It seems churlish to throw stones at these expensive psychedelic retreats. They aren't new. The wealthy have long cultivated a world of fancy rehab centres where celebrities and the uber-rich go to exorcise their addictions in luxury surrounds. Adding psychedelic medicine to the mix seems a logical next step, and unsurprising to see in Australia.

But where is the accessible future in all of this? It's fair to wonder whether psychedelic medicine is going to be something only afforded to the wealthiest members of the community. Maybe private health insurers start backing the therapy, but even then it will only be for their premium members.

But maybe it doesn't need to remain that way for too long. Maybe the paradigm of psychedelic medicine as we currently know it could be smashed open and reassembled into something new.

A BUG AND A BLIND

'I really hope that we're moving in a direction whereby we're looking at other models here, [that] we're not just looking at the most broken or the most pathologised groups, but that we could potentially look at this as a wellness thing,' says Marg Ross, who got Australia's first psychedelic trial going back in 2018.

There's that dirty word again. *Wellness*.

Marg Ross isn't the only psychologist working with psychedelics who brings up the 'w-word'. It comes up a lot. And every time it's mentioned, I feel myself flinch a little. My problem isn't with the word by itself, but with how wellness as a concept has been so thoroughly hijacked by pseudoscientific snake-oil salespeople that it feels disconcerting to think it the right place for psychedelics in Western society.

But that is the ideological space we end up in if we want to sit outside of the sick–well binary in Western medicine. You take medicine when you are sick. But what if you aren't 'sick' in the conventional sense?

Some people I spoke to were more pragmatic. Gill Bedi, for example, believes psychedelic medicine could be moved to earlier in our treatment processes. We're still going to a doctor and getting a diagnosis, but she doesn't see these drugs as a third-line or even fourth-line treatment. Psychotherapy, she believes, should always be the first port of call for most people, but it would be reasonable for a patient to quickly try some kind of psychedelic medicine instead of playing pinball with other antidepressant drugs.

I couldn't help but pose this question to myself. My own mental health issue was something that certainly didn't come on immediately. Even before that fateful 2023 trip to my GP, beginning the rollercoaster of antidepressants, I was a few years into what had been a noticeable decline.

Was there a point at which a well-timed and intentioned mushroom trip could have nudged me in a different direction? Or what if, instead of being given antidepressants as the first thing by my GP, I was forwarded to a new kind of clinic to have a quick dose of DMT one afternoon?

Almost every single conversation I had in the process of researching this book ended in the same place. I would ask whomever I was interviewing what they thought would be an ideal future for psychedelic medicine. And everyone ended up in some kind of imagined future where the fundamental way we do medicine was turned upside down. A future where we focused on prevention, catching people before they fall.

It dawned on me that most researchers, journalists and politicians have been asking the wrong questions for nearly a decade. This whole psychedelic medicine thing isn't about efficacy, or clinical targets. It's not about whether psychedelics *can heal*.

The real thorny question is: how can we best use psychedelics as a society, culture and community?

In my last conversation with Marg Ross, we really ended up in a strange rhetorical space. Ross is probably one of Australia's most experienced psychedelic clinicians but has been shifting her focus away from research towards real-world clinical practice. She firmly believes psychedelics do not lend themselves to our current clinical trial models. Despite finding powerful associations between psychedelics and clinical improvements in patients, Ross knows how mysterious these drugs fundamentally are.

When I asked Ross if she felt our current wave of psychedelic research is like trying to jam something into an ill-fitting container, she laughed warmly. The weirdness of psychedelics is the reason she thinks they are wonderful drugs, and yes, we are trying to hone away that novelty by turning them into a predictable medicine.

> I kind of love that [about psychedelics]. They're quite elusive that way. They're a bug and a blind. They frequently pose problems for researchers because they're so unpredictable. It's not like a usual medicine where we know that it's going to be this or it's going to be that. We've got the pharmacokinetics and the half-life data, but you really don't know what it's going to do.
>
> So there's a part of me that's quite delighted by that. But we must have a system that honours how these things work. If we're really going to work with this ... in medicine,

> in mental health, in wellbeing, we've got to come up with a different way of doing this. And I do think that doing it in community or doing it with others is going to be an important part of that.

And that was the kicker. Those words suddenly sent my mind spiralling through months of reading and research. It was like someone opened a search window in my brain and combed the database for the words 'community' and 'connection'.

Psychedelics haven't been used for thousands of years as a medicine to just make sick people well. More generally, psychoactive drugs have been used for thousands of years, by almost every culture, as a way of solidifying two things. Two things that, to me, seemed vitally important for a functional culture: community and connection.

MIX IN SOME BEER AND PARTY

If we want to consider things from the viewpoint of ancient use, modern psychedelic medicine is weird. We have turned psychedelics into a peculiar, solitary, internal exercise.

Take a drug. Put on headphones and an eye mask. Disassociate from your surroundings. Internalise the experience. Keep away from others. Find your trauma.

Despite any debate over the ways other cultures may have used these drugs in the past, it can be reasonably argued that the way 'we' are doing it – in the West, today – is a little bit different.

Anthropologist and religious scholar Des Tramacchi spent some time in the early 2000s drawing connections between modern Australian psychedelic parties (informally referred to as 'doofs') and various indigenous psychedelic rituals. One of his landmark articles, titled 'Entheogenic Dance Ecstasis', looked at several unifying factors linking Mexican peyote rituals, Amazonian yagé ceremonies and West African iboga rituals.[8] All these disparate ritual uses of psychedelics shared structural similarities, according to Tramacchi. This included consistent roles for music and dance.

Tramacchi argued the 'functional goal' of all these rituals was to 'renew and intensify group identification at an immediate level'. The fascinating way this is achieved is through an almost paradoxical alternation between internalising periods, going into the self, and externalising moments of shared 'community ecstasies'. In other words, there were parts of these rituals that resembled our modern medicalised psychedelic 'quest for the self' but they were never isolated from the collective ecstatic experience of the group. You can't do one without the other – both figuratively and literally.

And some more recent archaeological discoveries have suggested even broader ancient psychedelic uses beyond bonding just members of a single community. One of the most striking findings came in 2022, as part of a dig in northern Peru focusing on a group of people known as the Wari. Flourishing for a period of around 500 years, starting around 600 CE, the Wari were a fascinating people who were known to partake in an assortment of natural psychoactive substances.[9]

Of note was their use of a tree informally known as vilca. For a few months every year, this tree flowers, creating seed pods that contain two key psychedelic compounds: bufotenin and 5MeO-DMT. Archaeologists have found traces of vilca consumption in a variety of locations across South America but the Wari used it a little differently than others. Prior vilca discoveries were limited to specific archaeological spaces thought to be representative of use by an elite few in private ceremonial contexts. For the most part it was thought that vilca, usually smoked, was the province of a privileged few, possibly deployed as a way of affirming social hierarchy and control.

But this find in 2022 turned that idea on its head. Here, archaeologists found vilca seeds mixed up in the detritus of two other crops: maize and molle. Those crops were used to brew a beer-like alcoholic beverage known as chicha. The site also revealed chicha drinking vessels decorated with depictions of vilca seed pods. Something unusual was going on at this remote Wari outpost. The researchers found no trace of weaponry or any signs this was a military encampment. A strange hypothesis emerged. What if the Wari were 'spiking' their beer with psychedelics and holding big feast-like parties for local communities?

There were no vilca trees in the vicinity of the outpost. The hallucinogenic element to their special brews was likely a kind of secret knowledge. And the specific combination of hydrocarbons in the molle and the beta-carbolines arising from the fermentation process created a perfect environment to block those gut enzymes known to stop certain psychedelic molecules from being metabolised through the stomach. This allowed the psychedelic compounds from the vilca to have a minor effect when the beverage was drunk. It wouldn't have been anything like an out-of-body experience from smoking 5MeO-DMT, or a multi-hour interdimensional ayahuasca journey. Instead, it would have created a milder, more prosocial type of drunkenness. Perfect for making friends and influencing people.

The Wari discovery certainly isn't the only ancient use of psychedelics to demonstrate a more recreational mode of consumption. The Aztecs, for example, were known to use magic mushrooms in a variety of contexts, from priests eating them as a way of communing with gods to broader psychoactive mushroom feasting at big celebrations. One early Spanish missionary even reported magic mushrooms incorporated into human sacrifice rituals.[10] In fact, those being sacrificed may have been killed while under the influence of psychedelic mushrooms. The ultimate trip!

The big takeaway from this glimpse back in time is that psychoactive drugs were often used by cultures around the world as a way of cementing community, forging new social connections, and celebrating key collective moments. In contrast, our solipsistic modern medical model sidelines all those traditional uses, funnelling the drugs into a healing container solely focused on the self.

But so what? Psychedelics may work just fine for us as individual healing tools in the 21st century. Unless, of course, community and connection are two things that are disappearing from our modern world.

JOIN OR DIE

In the later years of the 20th century, American social scientist Robert Putnam randomly came across a piece of trivia in the newspaper. A local Parent Teacher Association (PTA) had falling membership numbers. Putnam was surprised; he had assumed every parent with a kid at school joined the PTA. Turns out that wasn't the case. PTA memberships across America were falling off a cliff. And it wasn't just school associations. Putnam quickly discovered general civic engagement across the board had been dropping since the 1970s – from church attendance and volunteering to union and club membership.

As Putnam started talking to colleagues about this odd situation, he mentioned to a friend one of his recent observations: a drop in membership of tenpin-bowling leagues. At this point in the early 1990s more people than ever were bowling, but across the prior 20 years the number of people who bowled in leagues had dropped by 40 per cent. The friend responded with surprise, saying to Putnam, 'My goodness, you mean they're bowling alone?'[11]

The random exclamation turned into the title of Putnam's first paper on the topic, published in 1995: 'Bowling Alone: America's Declining Social Capital'. The paper was a small outline of what would eventually become his magnum opus, a doorstopper of a political science book published in 2000.[12]

Being a social scientist with a view on political policy, Putnam's initial frame for the work was correlating this general decline of civic engagement with an increasingly dysfunctional democratic political system. His big idea emerged out of a massive real-world experiment he had been following for 25 years.

In 1970 Putnam was doing some boring political science work in Italy when he realised he was at the precipice of a grand natural experiment. The country had just undergone a profound governmental restructure – splitting up into around 20 smaller regional governments. Putnam saw the opportunity to accumulate a stunning body of data over the coming years, tracking which individual regional governments were successful and which weren't.

Over the next 20 years, Putnam managed to graph the most successful and least successful governments, looking at metrics such as how much a government achieved in terms of fulfilling its promises and how long a government stayed together, alongside qualitative data asking people how satisfied they were with their government. And then he tried to work out what environmental conditions corresponded with a government's success or failure.

Here came the massive surprise. You'd think education or wealth or urbanisation would be key factors at play but they weren't. Even evaluations of political polarisation didn't effectively track with a government's success or failure. Late in the project Putnam had a flash of inspiration. What about clubs? Social engagement? Thinking outside the box of politics, what did the data show about the way people in different regions connected with each other?

He aggregated a mass of data comparing rates of involvement in things like singing groups and sports clubs. He also rolled in data like newspaper readership and feelings of social trust. All this culminated in a new graph – a graph that rated the regions from least to most civically engaged.

And in a jaw-dropping eureka moment, Putnam saw this graph of civic engagement exactly matched the graph of government success. It was a magnificent achievement. He had uncovered something truly important, but what did it all mean? In his 1993 book *Making Democracy Work,* Putnam was still decoding his experiment. His description of those regions with low-levels of civic engagement is worth noting here, as the ripples of relevance to our world 30 years later are impossible to ignore:

> At the other pole are the 'uncivic' regions ... The very concept of 'citizen' here is stunted. From the point of view of the individual inhabitant, public affairs is the business of somebody else – *i notabili*, 'the bosses,' 'the politicians' – but not me ... Political participation is triggered by personal dependency or private greed, not by collective purpose. Engagement in social and cultural associations is meager ...
>
> Laws (almost everyone agrees) are made to be broken, but fearing others' lawlessness, people demand sterner discipline. Trapped in these interlocking vicious circles, nearly everyone feels powerless, exploited, and unhappy. All things considered, it is hardly surprising that representative government here is less effective than in more civic communities.[13]

Putnam's ideas about civic engagement, social connection and functional government were dropped into the world at the turn of the century, and other writers took the baton and ran. In 2010 writer-cum-politician Andrew Leigh adapted Putnam's ideas to an Australian context with his book *Disconnected.* Leigh effectively showed that all the same markers of decline that Putnam had noted could be traced in Australia. From the 1960s to the early 2000s, Australia saw most measures of 'social capital' decline:

> Organisational membership is down. We are less likely to attend church. Political parties and unions are bleeding members. Sporting participation and cultural attendance are down. Volunteering is most likely below its post-war peak, though it did record a rise in the late 1990s. We have fewer friends and are less connected with our neighbours than in the mid-1980s. Other measures have flatlined, but few have risen.[14]

The trend is growing even more pronounced. In February 2025 American journalist Derek Thompson pulled Putnam's ideas right up to the current moment in a thorough article titled 'The Anti-Social Century'.[15] Thompson dropped a heap of extra data on top of Putnam's, showing how technology has accelerated a decline in social connectedness. Since the turn of the century, Thompson argued, we have not only stopped participating in all the markers Putnam had measured as signs of healthy civic engagement, but we've also started dropping on a whole host of other interpersonal metrics. We have fewer friends than ever. We are going out less, staying home more. Real-life social networks have shrunk.

We are lonely.

And it's making us sick.

A MASSIVE 236-PAGE REPORT ON SOCIAL DISCONNECTION was published by the World Health Organization in mid-2025.[16] Consolidating scores of disparate studies into one big thesis, the report found around one in six people, across the entire world, had suffered some feeling of loneliness over the past decade. Those feeling social disconnection had higher rates of heart disease, stroke, depression and anxiety, and were dying younger than their less-lonely counterparts.

Of course, the relationship between all these factors is noted in almost every study as highly bidirectional. Someone with depression is likely to subsequently socialise less, for example, and that amplifies their mental health issues. Or loneliness may mean someone spends more time at home eating unhealthy food, leading to all the health problems that come with that.

But we can't wave this away as a mere bidirectional problem – everything causing everything. Some studies cited in the WHO report found people with highly social lives who drank and smoked tended not to have the same risk of death and disease as someone isolated, with few friends, but not smoking or drinking. Everything may be confounded, but there were distinct clues in the data showing loneliness and social isolation as powerfully detrimental to one's health.

We do know some things for sure. We know we are more divided, more lonely and more socially isolated, and have fewer friends than previous generations.

But what does this all have to do with psychedelics?

WE LIVE IN CHEMICAL RELATIONSHIPS

Why people are drawn to recreational uses of certain psychoactive substances can give us a clue about the kinds of benefits these substances may be offering. We know some ancient psychedelic uses encompassed ritual activities that solidified social bonds. These ceremonial uses often spanned multi-day events and included marathon intoxicated dance sessions. These shared experiences made a community stronger, cementing bonds that helped the culture both grow and defend itself from outside threats.

Looking to the early 1980s, for example, when MDMA began to leak out of its psychotherapy container into recreational uses, we immediately saw it emerge as a popular prosocial tonic among disco and nightclub patrons. The drug seemed to be an exceptional tool to potentiate a type of social bonding researchers have called 'identity fusion'.[17] This is a phenomenon where certain experiences lead to a kind of breakdown in the separation between the self and other. The more porous the border between me and you, the less we harbour feelings of disconnection and separation.

In 2017 a pair of anthropologists coined the term 'chemosociality' to describe the way drugs (or, more generally, chemicals) can catalyse bonds between people. The idea was deceptively simple. It suggested that 'longstanding relationships and emergent social forms [can] arise from chemical exposures and dependencies'.[18]

We can consider our lives dominated by chemosocial interactions, and once you begin to notice a few relationships mediated by chemicals, you start to see them everywhere. Bonds formed between cancer patients undergoing toxic chemotherapy. Passing encounters with particular friends over coffee. Celebratory connections mediated by alcohol. Anyone remember that whole episode of *Friends* based around the idea that smoking cigarettes together cements stronger relationships at work?

Drugs play crucial roles in a whole lot of our social engagements, and the idea of chemosocialities suggests these aren't just circumstantial accompaniments. Instead, the drugs themselves potentiate these bonds. Shared psychoactive experiences amplify connections between people.

Drawing this framework into the world of psychedelics was a paper published in 2023 from a trio of researchers we have already met: Tehseen Noorani, Gillinder Bedi and Suresh Muthukumaraswamy. The team provocatively suggested recent psychedelic clinical trials have been unduly influenced by chemosocial relationships. Their argument was that the social movements formed around modern psychedelic medicine have led to clinical trial results being overinflated.

That leaves researchers with three options. One: try to minimise the chemosocial effects of psychedelics so as to get more useful clinical trial data. Two: have each study attempt to document and measure the chemosocial influence in any individual trial.

The third option, however, is the one that really fascinates me. Instead of thinking about these chemosocial interactions as a bug to be eliminated, what if we consider them a valuable feature that we lean into? If one of the strengths of psychedelics is the way they cement feelings of connection, surely that is something that could help facilitate healing in whatever context is being tested?

The article cited a couple of clinical trials that looked to embrace the chemosocial properties of psychedelics. One trial, for example, set out to explore the effects of psilocybin accompanied by group therapy for older AIDS survivors suffering feelings of loss and demoralisation.[19] The drug-dosing days were all solo sessions, as with other modern medical uses, but the psychotherapy before and after was conducted in group contexts. The cohort was also encouraged to share contact details and meet outside of the group therapy sessions. All this was geared at enhancing what the trial noted as 'group cohesion'.

If we really want to think outside of the box, we need to decimate some paradigms. Maybe the best way to integrate psychedelics into our culture involves breaking the drugs out of the solitary medical mould. But how would we do that?

THE POLLINATION APPROACH

One of the most fascinating speculative, future-focused paradigm shifts I've come across is an idea called the Pollination Approach. Conceived by US economist Bennet Zelner, the idea is based on the belief that one of the beneficial aspects of psychedelic use is the way the drug opens a window to community connection. Zellner's idea is to draw psychedelic medicine out of pharmaceutical systems and re-situate it in community spaces. To do this he proposes an interconnected network of 'psychedelic community wellness centres'. These are spaces that ostensibly serve as psychedelic clinics, where people go and experience these medicines in safe, therapeutically directed environments. But these spaces are far from cold, clinical spaces; they also serve as community hubs for a broad assortment of other services.

Each psychedelic centre is locally owned, and run by members of the community. Psychedelics are thus turned into tools that can serve individual health or wellness outcomes while also connecting and building community. It's undoubtedly a utopian vision, but it's not one entirely divorced from a sense of pragmatic reality. An example Zelner often cites of the way community can be integrated into medicine is the story of a small town in the UK called Frome.

In 2013 a doctor in Frome was struck with just how many patients she saw that were suffering from an underlying sense of loneliness and disconnection. A wonderful experiment was launched, called the Compassionate Frome Project. The idea was to connect patients who had complex social needs to a larger network of community groups. When a patient presented to a

GP, they were subsequently linked with people called 'community connectors'. These were volunteers trained to help patients find broad support within the community.

More than 400 groups and organisations were integrated into the system, helping people with everything from managing their finances to exercising better. Some people were linked up with choir groups or writing workshops, while others were connected with local charities.

Four years later the results came in, and they were stunning.[20] Compared to other towns across the county of Somerset, Frome saw emergency hospital admissions drop by 17 per cent. The rest of Somerset had tracked a 29 per cent increase in emergency admissions over the same period. Most of Somerset recorded a 21 per cent spike in general health costs while Frome reported a 21 per cent drop in similar costs.

Zelner sees the Frome story as a good example of how modern medical systems can be embedded into local communities. And it's not difficult to imagine a way his Pollination model could morph into something like the Frome system.

A more psychedelically focused future paradigm can be seen in the newly implemented Natural Medicine Health Act in the American state of Colorado. As a piecemeal array of different state-based measures for psychedelic drug access spread across the United States, Colorado's approach stands out. Systems in the state were built to create regulated healing centres, but alongside this the state wholly decriminalised psilocybin, DMT and mescaline. The decrim program was clear and comprehensive. Adults over the age of 21 could cultivate, possess and consume these substances. And the legislation went even further: a sharing rule was legislated, allowing the substances to be passed between adults under the proviso that no money changed hands.

As of 2026 the Colorado system is only just coming online, following a few years of regulatory development. It's not clear how this experiment will play out but the framework is open to an optimistic kind of psychedelic community club model. The idea would be that community centres emerge to serve as information and distribution hubs for psychedelics.

Join a club, find your people, take the trip, make some connections.

A NARROW RENAISSANCE

In early 2024 I interviewed clinical psychologist Rosalind Watts for a story investigating how some pharmaceutical companies were working to remove psychotherapy from their psychedelic medicine treatment protocol. Watts had worked on an early UK clinical trial on psilocybin for depression before becoming disillusioned with the way modern psychedelic medicine was going.

She felt patients were being given these drugs with nowhere near the amount of social support necessary. Her experiences in these trials revealed many patients struggled with integrating their psychedelic revelations into their normal lives. As soon as the trial period ended, a portion of participants almost always were left struggling to cope.

One thing Watts said to me in that interview really stuck with me. 'If you put psychedelics into a disconnected culture, then people go back to disconnectedness, and they're left with these big, huge questions and no one to talk to.'

It was a thought that kept rising to the surface as I was working on this book. And it was a thought echoed in many conversations I had with current psychedelic practitioners. As Marg Ross said to me, the biggest issue she faced in her psilocybin clinical trial was participants feeling a deep need to share their experiences with others.

'One of my biggest learnings from the study was that people came out of this and have profound experiences – profound. But there was an isolation in that, because they didn't know who else they could speak to aside from us as the therapists. If they wanted to talk to anyone about it, they felt like they were going to sound crazy,' Ross told me. 'And that was my greatest regret ... I didn't have a group where they could come and talk about their experiences, and feel that they [could] speak openly.' Participants yearned for a connection with others, and it was a connection that the researchers were unable to offer within the strict parameters of a clinical trial.

Alongside that recurring observation, there was another constant and discordant story emerging among those who were working with psychedelics. The personal experiences that led people to believe in the potential of these drugs were experiences that involved social or recreational uses. Some may have encountered psychedelics with intention – participating in a healing-focused ayahuasca ceremony, for example – but they mostly weren't suffering the kind of deep-seated, treatment-resistant mental health conditions that modern medicine has been focusing on.

The most pertinent example of this contradiction is also probably the most potent.

German billionaire Christian Angermayer is about as straight-edge as they come, reportedly not even drinking a sip of alcohol in the first 30 years of his life. A big pharmaceutical investor, he heard about the supposed benefits of psychedelics back in 2013. The next year he happened to be with friends yachting in the Caribbean when the option of taking some magic mushrooms arose. So Angermayer had his first psychedelic experience, with friends on a beach in the Caribbean, and he found it to be 'hands down the single most important, moving, deepest thing I've ever done'.[21]

Being an entrepreneurial person, Angermayer quickly thought – and this is a direct quote – 'How can I make a business out of this?' Within a few years Angermayer, along with other billionaires including Peter Thiel, had founded the big landmark psychedelic pharma companies pushing to make the drugs commercial medicines, including atai Life Sciences, now AtaiBeckley (working with DMT and 5MeO-DMT) and Compass Pathways (working with psilocybin). These powerful corporations are laser-focused on turning psychedelics into patented medicines.

Many a billionaire's psychedelic advocacy story begins with a recreational mushroom trip on the beach. The irony should be clear. 'Taking these drugs with friends on a beach may have delivered incredible experiences to me, but I'll not be working to help others freely or legally have those same experiences,' our billionaire might think. 'Instead, what I can do is turn these things into controllable, marketable and profitable medicines, at the same time limiting any of the broader uses that got me interested in all of this in the first place.'

The big 21st-century 'psychedelic renaissance' we love to talk about is barely a renaissance. Maybe in the beginning it promised something bigger, when Rick Strassman was doing his wild research with DMT, or early Johns Hopkins researchers were exploring mystical experiences with psilocybin. But over the last decade, that kind of research has dwindled. The lane has narrowed, and medicinal development now drives all study. Big money with a laser focus; that's the name of the psychedelic science game in the 2020s. What medicines can we make? What evidence do we need to gather for regulators? How can we roll the new drugs out and make some money?

Perhaps the real problem here is the commercialisation of psychedelics. Not only is all research winnowing into pharmaceutical company channels, but there's an idea that turning these drugs into medical treatments we pay money for generates an expectation of having our problems solved – for a price. Informally, I've already heard stories of this surfacing as a problem in the few instances of patients being legally treated in the Australian model. There may have been barely 100 patients treated so far in the new Australian system; for some of them, this therapy didn't work. And these patients are not happy.

I mean, I can't blame them. If I'd consumed years of evangelical news stories about the miracle of psychedelics and then paid $30 000 to have my PTSD or depression treated, I would expect it to work. Hell, maybe I'd even demand it work.

AT THE END OF ALL THIS RESEARCH AND WRITING, I'D hoped to be able to offer a kind of pithy yet positive conclusion. 'This is what we should be working towards,' I'd suggest, summing up the entire book in a cute, punchy paragraph. But after working on this for a couple of years, I realise I have no simple answers.

Things are going in a certain medicalised direction. I'm sure these drugs will be squeezed into our medical models in some contorted way over the tail end of the 2020s. However ill-fitting this may be, it is happening.

And don't get me wrong – this is not a bad thing. These drugs will help some people who have been struggling with uncontrolled mental health conditions. Some patients will find profound relief. Lives will be saved by introducing new, albeit not widely accessible, treatments. Every clinician working with these drugs has recounted stories of patients experiencing transformative healing after years of suffering. Psychedelics can, and likely will, be wonderful medicines for some people.

If I silence the cynic in me, I can almost hear an optimistic voice advocating the Trojan Horse model: suggesting this initial stage of medicalisation is just the first step towards a more integrated, community-focused psychedelic future. The idea is that once we let these drugs out into the wild, they can't – they won't – be contained. Give it a few years and treatment protocols will broaden, access will widen.

But the cynic is louder, struggling to see how our clinical uses become cheaper, or more accessible, without safety measures being skirted and looser clinicians offering treatments in dangerous ways. Maybe AI-driven therapy models will be developed to make things more scalable (as if this is a good thing – tripping with ChatGPT). And blending more entrepreneurial or profitable protocols with patented psychedelic medicines doesn't exactly pave the way for us to connect better with one another. We've done all this work and ended up with a few new medicines that doctors can prescribe for those who are extremely ill.

I'm not an activist. I'm not an advocate. I'm not an evangelist. I'm a journalist. And all my work following the movement of psychedelics in science and medicine over the years has led me to sincerely believe these substances have some beneficial uses – medical and otherwise. They can change some people's lives for the better. But is boxing psychedelics into a tightly controlled medical container the only way we can think of using these drugs? Can we learn something from the way other cultures around the world have used drugs in the past? And what, really, do we need right now to help our world be better?

Making a few new medicines can't be the *only* way we use psychedelics.

Surely there are other ways.

EPILOGUE

November 2025. The first Entheogenesis Australis (EGA) outdoor event in eight years happened to coincide with Victoria's wettest November in decades. Everything was a little different but still familiar. For me the biggest change was attending the event with a tiny three-and-a-half-year-old human being attached to my leg. I'd known the EGA folk since the organisation's genesis 21 years before. The lifespan of this event crossed paths with a weird assortment of different versions of me over the years.

Early on Monday morning, after a hectic weekend of hosting, chatting and parenting, I groggily went to the kitchen in one of the crew cabins to make a coffee; caffeine was the drug I needed. A friend was sitting at the table, tapping away at his laptop and grumbling about an email problem. We were plugging back in to the matrix after a wonderful 48 hours of digital disconnection. I pulled my phone out and began the requisite zombie scroll.

And boy, did the algorithm deliver. The first thing that jumped out of my feed was an ongoing global livestream event. A billionaire in the United States was streaming, in real time, a high-dose magic-mushroom experience. The tripper I was watching was none other than Bryan Johnson, the 'don't die' entrepreneur obsessed with living forever. He'd recently leaped on a research article that suggested psilocybin could have longevity properties, and now he was testing it out for himself (in a supposedly legal, albeit undisclosed, location and context).

The moment I tuned in was about as surreal as it gets. In one corner of the screen, Johnson lay on a mat, curled up, with an eye mask on. Three other men filled the rest of the screen talking about things like what we can do to prevent epigenetic aging and how psychedelics apparently kickstarted civilisation back in ancient Greece. It was a bit like a dumb, bizarro version of the presentations I'd been watching in real life all weekend. Except instead of experts, scientists, academics and people who knew what they were talking about, I soon found out these three guys were simply millionaire tech investors and entrepreneurs.

Later, Grimes played a live DJ set over Zoom to bring Johnson out of the deepest part of his trip. At one point in the set, Johnson's partner (in business and life) held up a sign saying, 'Grimes, he's loving this, we love you'. A touching moment indeed.

The whole thing was a perfect synthesis of psychedelic culture in the mid-2020s. A billionaire doing shrooms alone in a room, joined by an assortment of his wealthy friends on Zoom, all telecast to an international audience of thousands on X and YouTube. The performative nature of the whole enterprise was head-spinning. Johnson gave the impression, especially in the lead-up to the event, that this was an all-new experience for him. He never explicitly said this was to be his first psychedelic experience, or even his first magic-mushroom experience, but that was certainly the impression most people received. And so thousands of people tuned in to see if a billionaire capitalist entrepreneur was about to be humbled by the power of magic mushrooms. Was Johnson about to take psychedelics and realise all his previous beliefs were wrong? The mushroom medicine was going to tell him to give all his money away, stop being selfish, and help save the world?

Of course not.

What Johnson cleverly kept out of the limelight in the lead-up to this six-hour livestreamed advertisement for something was that he was far from psychedelically naive. It's unclear whether he'd had significant magic-mushroom experiences in the past, but it turns out he was a massive fan and proselytiser of 5MeO-DMT – so much that he even had a tattoo of the molecule on his body. We weren't watching someone innocently experience psychedelics for the first time. This was a guy intimately familiar with the most powerful psychedelic molecule on the planet playacting the 'whirlwind' of a mushroom experience, from masked internalisation to late-trip giggly sincerity.

I'd just spent the weekend talking about psychedelics, science, consciousness, everything, with some of the cleverest people I'd ever met. Real-life conversations. Face to face, in all the fleshy discomfort of a real-world space. It was exciting, rejuvenating and real. A reminder of the value in genuine interpersonal connection.

And now I was watching this: a crass, disconnected, performative thing on my phone. Who is steering the direction of the psychedelic renaissance again?

This 2025 EGA event felt like another landmark juncture; perhaps, like prior events, it won't really be clear what it means until we look back in hindsight. In the moment there was undoubtedly a shift in the tenor of the event. Back in 2010 we'd felt electricity at the prospect of MDMA becoming legitimised in a world where it was considered nothing more than an illicit recreational drug that damages your body and brain. By 2017 it was serious business. Psychedelics were coming out of the closet and discussions were all about how to shepherd these things into mainstream consciousness.

In 2025, however, the mood was different. Excitement was tempered. Maybe even something like confusion was the predominant sensation. The path to medicalisation was certainly underway, but for many at the event there was an overriding feeling of 'Now what?'

Massive pharmaceutical companies were paying billions of dollars to license psychedelic drugs, both new and old. Powerful market forces had taken the reins of research and development. Any pre-existing hopes for broader decriminalisation efforts were being efficiently quashed.

Alongside this, I left the 2025 event with some vague concerns. Modern psychedelic psychotherapy seemed to be celebrating the idea it was secular, devoid of ideological interference. But that wasn't really what I had seen, in the years of reporting on psychedelic medicine, and in my decades of being around psychedelic folk.

We think we've created a medical container for psychedelics that is neutral (as if neutrality is a noble goal in and of itself). We are wary of creating spaces that could unduly influence the beliefs of patients, so the modern psychedelic experience valorises autonomy. We are told to internalise the experience, listen to 'the self', and trust that whatever surfaces is what your body needs to resolve in order to heal. The method has frequently been described to me as 'non-directive'. The therapist is framed more like a midwife than a surgeon. Words like 'facilitation' and 'guidance' are used, and the paradigm of the inner healer is proffered.

But is this model *really* neutral?

It *seems* like we have constructed an approach for using psychedelics that is devoid of external suggestion. No values are being forced on the patient, no world view imposed. It's all coming from inside you.

Except that is its own bias, and not so coincidentally it's also a value system entirely in sync with modern Western sensibilities. Psychedelic medicine in the 21st century privileges the individual. We have found a way to contain the weirdness of psychedelics, hone away any sharp edges, remove communal complications, and create a model of healing that is infatuated with the self.

My online algorithm has become so confused by all the psychedelic research I do that I now have a front-row seat to every alternative psychology and psychedelic advertisement you can imagine. As I write this I see an ad for an ayahuasca retreat suggesting 'the medicine' is a door to 'our truest self'. Again, this constant focus on finding your self. Ayn Rand would be so proud to see how the psychedelic world has embraced her philosophies.

Find your self?

Shouldn't we be reconnecting with others?

How about *finding* the others?

There's a popular story about Timothy Leary – again, perhaps it's apocryphal. He is giving a talk, and afterwards, during the Q&A, a woman stands up and says, 'I've had psychedelics. I get it. I've seen the world is connected. But what do I do now?' Leary responds with a short, three-word answer.

'Find the others.'

The sentiment was elegant in its simplicity. Leary was suggesting we need to find our tribe, our people. If you have any kind of novel experience, you must get out into the world and find those who can relate to you. This is how we build our tribe.

It's an admirable sentiment, and likely one that was of great use in the mid-to-late 20th century. A clarion call to all the weirdos and freaks. Find your people. Join forces. Make your power.

Of course, now, in the wild west of the 21st century's polarised hyper-tribalism, I'm not so sure the sentiment is helpful. And neither was media theorist and cultural commentator Douglas Rushkoff.

I interviewed Rushkoff in 2023 and talked to him about this Leary quote. For many, Rushkoff had become a spiritual successor to Leary. He wrote prolifically about counterculture, technology and psychedelics in the 1990s. And then, as the new millennium dawned, he began to chronicle how technology was being coopted by oppressive commercial forces. He reimagined Leary's 'find the others' call.

Rushkoff quite correctly saw our modern world as beset by tribalism. Social media algorithms not only helped us find *our others* but they weaponised that feeling of 'us versus them'. So he turned the saying on its head. What we need to do now, he suggested, was find the *others*. Cross the ideological divide. Talk to those with differing beliefs. Get to that common ground.

To Rushkoff, our disassociation required reconciliation. It needed people to meet in the middle, and for both sides to remember that we're all still kinda the same.

I liked the idea. And I liked the way it turned Leary's original call on its head. But thinking about where the world is right now, I'm not sure that simply crossing the divide and chatting with 'the others' is what we need. In the 2020s, civil discourse has become a game in which someone sits under a banner proclaiming 'Prove me wrong', facing off in a war of words with those of differing beliefs.

Post-Covid, we are more alone than ever. We've gone from bowling alone to tripping alone, or even just watching people trip alone on livestreams. Our existence is increasingly virtual. Work is remote. Conversations are group threads on our phones dominated by memes and gifs. I yell into the void on whatever social media platform has become my identity – oh, you're a LinkedIn person; I like Bluesky. That guy is still on Facebook? The kids are back on Snapchat?

So here is my take on the Leary/Rushkoff call-out.

I say: find one another.

We need to re-enter the meatspace. It's simpler than anything Rushkoff or Leary suggested, and perhaps that makes it an indictment of our times, but here we are. The need is not complicated. Share space with others. Any others – it doesn't matter.

Find one another.

For thousands of years, people have used psychoactive substances to solidify social bonds. Sharing a drink, a smoke, a mushroom, or just a dance. The altered state of consciousness doesn't necessarily need to be generated by a drug. As we've found, a whole host of experiences can work to tune people together. Of course, drugs are pretty effective, but this is far from a paean to drug use.

Instead, the point here is to get away from the digital space and into a real communal environment. Connection is the thing of import. Psychedelics fuel connection, and that's one of the big things missing from modern psychedelic medicine, but the benefits come from the connections, not the drugs. I'm trying to silence my inner cynic. Quieten down the misanthrope. Settle the outrage. I know what we have to do.

Find one another.

NOTES

Introduction

1 Jay, M. (2018). Bicycle day revisited. *Mike Jay*. https://mikejay.net/bicycle-day-revisited/

2 Bender, D. A., Dunn, H. M., Pekau, A., Mohite, A. D., Anandarajah, A., Ross, B. D., Steinle, J., Shankar, S., Kiley, B., Martin, S., Gonuguntla, R., Stonov, M., Pippala, N., Abdalla, R., Stille, M. K., Yusuf, J., Villalba, M., Werner, G., Divekar, A., Daniels-Tineo, M., … Nemeroff, C. B. (2026). Trends in the psychedelic renaissance: Applying artificial intelligence to measure media portrayal of psychedelic drugs in the 21st century. *BJPsych Open, 12*(2), e63. https://doi.org/10.1192/bjo.2025.10974

3 Haridy, R. (2023, March 26). How to write a psychedelic renaissance news story. *Rich Haridy*. https://www.richharidy.com/blog/how-to-write-a-psychedelic-renaissance-news-story

4 Robb, A. (2019, November 21). Richard Nixon's 'war on drugs' claims casualties every day. *The Australian*. https://www.theaustralian.com.au/commentary/richard-nixons-war-on-drugs-claims-casualties-every-day/news-story/db75a2d102c58f03ca02bfd6b466a9d5?amp

5 Kupferschmidt, K. (2016, December 1). Hallucinogenic drugs help cancer patients deal with their fear of death. *Science*. https://www.science.org/content/article/hallucinogenic-drugs-help-cancer-patients-deal-their-fear-death

6 Tanne J. H. (2004). Humphry Osmond. *BMJ: British Medical Journal, 328*(7441), 713. https://doi.org/10.1136/bmj.328.7441.713; Ostrand, A., Nour, M., Timmermann, C., Rosati, A., Luan, L. X., Gómez-Emilsson, A. G., Bornemann, J., Greenway, K., Roseman, L., & Carhart-Harris, R. (2025, December 4). Defining 'psychedelic' [preprint]. https://www.researchgate.net/publication/398347750_Defining_'psychedelic'

7 Ostrand et al. (2025). Defining 'psychedelic'.

1 History

1 Evelyn was interviewed by researcher and historian Jonathan Carmichael in 2023. The interview is unpublished. I am deeply grateful the material has been shared and, with Evelyn's permission, published in this book.

2 Roberts, A. (2025). *Albion dreaming: A popular history of LSD in Britain* (2nd ed.). Psychedelic Press, p. 32.

3 Sandison, R. A., Spencer, A. M., & Whitelaw, J. D. A. (1954). The therapeutic value of lysergic acid diethylamide in mental illness, *Journal of Mental Science, 100*(419), 491–507. https://doi.org/10.1192/bjp.100.419.491

4 Whitaker, L. H. (1964). Lysergic acid diethylamide in psychotherapy. I: Clinical aspects. *Medical Journal of Australia, 1,* 5–8.

5 Passie, T., Guss, J., & Krähenmann, R. (2022). Lower-dose psycholytic therapy – A neglected approach. *Frontiers in Psychiatry, 13,* 1020505. https://doi.org/10.3389/fpsyt.2022.1020505

6 Passie et al. (2022). Lower-dose psycholytic therapy.

7 Passie et al. (2022). Lower-dose psycholytic therapy.

8 Passie et al. (2022). Lower-dose psycholytic therapy.

9 Whitaker (1964). Lysergic acid diethylamide ... Part I.

10 Whitaker (1964). Lysergic acid diethylamide ... Part I.

11 Whitaker (1964). Lysergic acid diethylamide ... Part I; Whitaker, L. H. (1964). Lysergic acid diethylamide in psychotherapy. Part II: Results. *Medical Journal of Australia, 1,* 36–41.

12 Oram, M. (2018). *The trials of psychedelic therapy: LSD psychotherapy in America.* Johns Hopkins University Press. https://dx.doi.org/10.1353/book.60680.

13 Miller, M. T. (1991). Thalidomide embryopathy: A model for the study of congenital incomitant horizontal strabismus. *Transactions of the American Ophthalmological Society, 89,* 623–674.

14 Rensberger, B. (1975, July 12). C.I.A. in the early nineteen-fifties was among pioneers in research on L.S.D.'s effects. *New York Times.* https://www.nytimes.com/1975/07/12/archives/cia-in-the-early-nineteenfifties-was-among-pioneers-in-research-on.html; Jarnow, J. (2016, October 6). LSD now: How the psychedelic renaissance changed acid. *Rolling Stone.* https://www.rollingstone.com/feature/lsd-now-how-the-psychedelic-renaissance-changed-acid-115775/; Pollan, M. (2019). *How to change your mind: The new science of psychedelics.* Penguin Books; Carhart-Harris, R.L., & Goodwin, G. M. (2017). The therapeutic potential of psychedelic drugs: Past, present, and future. *Neuropsychopharmacology, 42*(11), 2105–2113. https://doi.org/10.1038/npp.2017.84

15 Lomax, M. K. (2017). *Beyond the aetiology debate: The 'great LSD scandal' at Newhaven Private Hospital & the social foundations of mental health legislation in Victoria, Australia* [Doctoral dissertation, University of Melbourne]. University of Melbourne Library. https://hdl.handle.net/11343/208997

16 Lomax (2017). *Beyond the aetiology,* p. 171.

17 There are conflicting accounts of when Whitaker first met Anne. It was either 1963 or 1964, depending on the source. From my reporting, 1964, the date referenced by researcher Megan Lomax in her thesis, seems more likely; the timeline for the other events, such as Evelyn's growing suspicions, match up a little more effectively.

18 Johnston, C., & Jones, R. (2017). *The Family.* Scribe Publications, 'Sacred Manna' chapter.

19 Johnston & Jones (2017). *The Family.*

20 Johnston & Jones (2017). *The Family.*

21 Johnston & Jones (2017). *The Family.*

22 Zoates, T. (2017, February 19). Escape from 'The Family'. *Toby the Punk Poofy Cat*. https://tobyzoates.blogspot.com/2017/02/escape-from-family.html. Toby Zoates has published a detailed account of his time at Newhaven across several posts on his blog.

23 Zoates (2017). Escape from 'The Family'.

24 Lomax (2017). *Beyond the aetiology*, p. 174.

25 Lomax, *Beyond the aetiology*, pp. 183–184.

26 Lomax, *Beyond the aetiology*, pp. 31–32.

27 This estimate is a ballpark figure. The only definitive recorded number of patients treated in Australia with psychedelics came in a survey conducted by the Royal Australian and New Zealand College of Psychiatrists in 1970. That survey tracked 11 of the 19 authorised psychiatrists in Victoria, and found that around 4000 patients had been treated to that point. A report in *The Age* from 1991 suggests 'thousands' more patients were treated in that same period by the other eight authorised psychiatrists, and thousands more patients were likely treated in the unsurveyed period from 1970 to 1975. So a rough figure of 10 000 is reasonable.

28 Johnston & Jones (2017). *The Family*.

29 Strauss, N. (n.d.). *A psychedelic diary*. Nigel Strauss. https://nigelstrauss.com.au/books

30 McArthur, G. (2019, January 14). Magic mushroom therapy trial for terminally ill. *Herald Sun*. https://www.heraldsun.com.au/news/victoria/magic-mushroom-therapy-trial-for-terminally-ill/news-story/719909e03eaecad63473dacac0b272a6

31 Hunt, G. (2021, March 17). $15 million for development of innovative therapies for mental illness. [Media release]. Australian Government Department of Health and Aged Care. https://www.health.gov.au/ministers/the-hon-greg-hunt-mp/media/15-million-for-development-of-innovative-therapies-for-mental-illness

32 Ross, M. L., Iyer, R., Williams, M. L., Boughey, M., O'Callaghan, C., Hiscock, R., & Dwyer, J. (2025). Psilocybin-assisted psychotherapy for depression and anxiety associated with life threatening illness: A phase 2b randomized controlled trial. *General Hospital Psychiatry, 96*, 322–331. https://doi.org/10.1016/j.genhosppsych.2025.08.001

2 Magic mushrooms

1 This is the very first published description of a psychedelic magic mushroom experience in Australia.

2 Jamieson, A. (2025, August 13). *Finding into death without inquest … Rachael Lee Dixon*. COR 2024 002097. Coroner's Court of Victoria. https://www.coronerscourt.vic.gov.au/inquests-findings/findings

3 Woman's Day. (2025, April 2). Mushroom victim Rachael Dixon's sister: 'We still want answers'. *Woman's Day* (NZ). https://www.nowtolove.co.nz/news/rachael-dixon-mushroom-death/

4 Woman's Day (2025). Mushroom victim Rachael Dixon's sister.

5 Jamieson (2025). *Finding into death without inquest*, pp. 5–7.
6 Marks, J. (1979). *The search for the 'Manchurian candidate': The CIA and mind control.* Times Books, pp. 105–121. https://archive.org/details/searchformanchur00john/page/104/mode/2up
7 Hofmann, A. (1980). *LSD: My problem child* (J. Ott, Trans.). McGraw-Hill, ch. 6. (Original work published 1979.) https://maps.org/images/pdf/books/lsdmyproblemchild.pdf
8 Agurell, S., & Nilsson, J. L. (1968). A biosynthetic sequence from tryptophan to psilocybin. *Tetrahedron Letters, 9*, 1063–1064. https://doi.org/10.1016/S0040-4039(01)98891-4
9 Yokoyama, K. (1973). Poisoning by a hallucinogenic mushroom, Psilocybe subcaerulipes Hongo. *Transactions of the Mycological Society of Japan, 14*(3), 317–320.
10 Allen, J. W., Merlin, M. D., & Jansen, K. L. (1991). An ethnomycological review of psychoactive agarics in Australia and New Zealand. *Journal of Psychoactive Drugs, 23*(1), 39–69. https://doi.org/10.1080/02791072.1991.10472573
11 Allen et al. (1991). An ethnomycological review.
12 Stamets, P. (1996). *Psilocybin mushrooms of the world: An identification guide.* Ten Speed Press.
13 Notapillow. (2009, February 19). Mushroom paralysis (wood lovers) [Online forum post]. *Shroomery.* https://www.shroomery.org/forums/showflat.php/Number/9830137/fpart/1/vc/1
14 Notapillow, Mushroom paralysis (wood lovers).
15 This date was only affirmed in late 2023 when a team of biologists tracked psilocybin genes back using the largest magic mushroom genetic dataset ever gathered. Bradshaw, A. J., Ramírez-Cruz, V., Awan, A. R., Furci, G., Guzmán-Dávalos, L., & Dentinger, B. T. M. (2024). Phylogenomics of the psychoactive mushroom genus *Psilocybe* and evolution of the psilocybin biosynthetic gene cluster. *Proceedings of the National Academy of Sciences of the United States of America, 121*(3), e2311245121. https://doi.org/10.1073/pnas.2311245121
16 Longrich, N. R., Scriberas, J., & Wills, M. A. (2016). Severe extinction and rapid recovery of mammals across the Cretaceous–Palaeogene boundary, and the effects of rarity on patterns of extinction and recovery. *Journal of Evolutionary Biology, 29*(8), 1495–1512. https://doi.org/10.1111/jeb.12882
17 Bardeen, C. G., Garcia, R. R., Toon, O. B., & Conley, A. J. (2017). On transient climate change at the Cretaceous–Paleogene boundary due to atmospheric soot injections. *Proceedings of the National Academy of Sciences, 114*(36), E7415–E7424. https://doi.org/10.1073/pnas.1708980114
18 Potter, L. (2024). *Psychoactive psilocybin's evolution in 'magic mushrooms'.* University of Utah. https://attheu.utah.edu/facultystaff/psychoactive-psilocybins-evolution-in-magic-mushrooms/

19 Oss, O. T., & Oeric, O. N. (1991). *Psilocybin: Magic mushroom grower's guide* (rev. ed.). Quick American Publishing. http://www.psilosophy.info/resources/Psilocybin.magic.mushroom.growers.guide.pdf

20 Lenz, C., Sherwood, A., Kargbo, R., & Hoffmeister, D. (2021). Taking different roads: L-tryptophan as the origin of psilocybe natural products. *ChemPlusChem, 86*(1), 28–35. https://doi.org/10.1002/cplu.202000581

21 Fricke, J., Blei, F., & Hoffmeister, D. (2017). Enzymatic synthesis of psilocybin. *Angewandte Chemie International Edition, 56*(40), 12352–12355. https://doi.org/10.1002/anie.201705489

22 McTaggart, A. R., McLaughlin, S., Slot, J. C., McKernan, K., Appleyard, C., Bartlett, T. L., Weinert, M., Barlow, C., Warne, L. N., Shuey, L. S., Drenth, A., & James, T. Y. (2023). Domestication through clandestine cultivation constrained genetic diversity in magic mushrooms relative to naturalized populations. *Current Biology, 33*(23). https://doi.org/10.1016/j.cub.2023.10.059

23 *Azure* and *cyan* are both words for colours in the blue spectrum. In fact, *subaeruginosa* is also a word with origins in a Latin word meaning 'bluish'. As well as sharing visual similarities, these mushrooms are known for the way they stain blue when bruised.

24 McTaggart, A. R., Scarlettt, K., Slot, J. C., Barlow, C., Appleyard, C., Gardiner, D. M., Fechner, N., Tilden, J., Hass, D., Voogelbreinder, S., Lording, W. J., Lloyd, R. A., Shuey, L. S., Drenth, A., & James, T. Y. (2024). Wood-loving magic mushrooms from Australia are saprotrophic invaders in the Northern Hemisphere. *Fungal Systematics and Evolution, 14*(1), 209–222. https://doi.org/10.3114/fuse.2024.14.14

25 Ben-Shabat, S., Fride, E., Sheskin, T., Tamiri, T., Rhee, M. H., Vogel, Z., Bisogno, T., De Petrocellis, L., Di Marzo, V., & Mechoulam, R. (1998). An entourage effect: Inactive endogenous fatty acid glycerol esters enhance 2-arachidonoyl-glycerol cannabinoid activity. *European Journal of Pharmacology, 353*(1), 23–31. https://doi.org/10.1016/S0014-2999(98)00392-6

26 Simei, J. L. Q., Souza, J. D. R., Lisboa, J. R., Campos, A. C., Guimarães, F. S., Zuardi, A., & Crippa, J. A. S. (2024). Does the 'entourage effect' in cannabinoids exist? A narrative scoping review. *Cannabis and Cannabinoid Research, 9*(5), 1202–1216. https://doi.org/10.1089/can.2023.0052

27 Christensen, C., Rose, M., Cornett, C., & Allesø, M. (2023). Decoding the postulated entourage effect of medicinal cannabis: What it is and what it isn't. *Biomedicines, 11*(8), 2323. https://doi.org/10.3390/biomedicines11082323

28 Cogan, P. S. (2020). The 'entourage effect' or 'hodge-podge hashish': The questionable rebranding, marketing, and expectations of cannabis polypharmacy. *Expert Review of Clinical Pharmacology, 13*(8), 835–845. https://doi.org/10.1080/17512433.2020.1721281

29 Bauer, B. E. (2019, April 1). Wood lover paralysis from magic mushrooms: The aeruginascin hypothesis. *Psychedelic Science Review.*

https://psychedelicreview.com/wood-lover-paralysis-from-magic-mushrooms-the-aeruginascin-hypothesis/

30 Gartz, J. (1989). Analysis of aeruginascin in fruit bodies of the mushroom Inocybe aeruginascens. *International Journal of Crude Drug Research, 27*(3), 141–144. https://doi.org/10.3109/13880208909053954

31 Gartz (1989). Analysis of aeruginascin.

32 Lenz, C., Wick, J., & Hoffmeister, D. (2017). Identification of ω-*N*-methyl-4-hydroxytryptamine (norpsilocin) as a psilocybe natural product. *Journal of Natural Products, 80*(10), 2835–2838. https://doi.org/10.1021/acs.jnatprod.7b00407

33 Rakoczy, R. J., Runge, G. N., Sen, A. K., Sandoval, O., Wells, H. G., Nguyen, Q., Roberts, B. R., Sciortino, J. H., Gibbons, W. J.Jr, Friedberg, L. M., Jones, J. A., & McMurray, M. S. (2024). Pharmacological and behavioural effects of tryptamines present in psilocybin-containing mushrooms. *British Journal of Pharmacology, 181*(19), 3627–3641. https://doi.org/10.1111/bph.16466

34 Winter, C. A., & Flataker, L. (1956). Effects of lysergic acid diethylamide upon performance of trained rats. *Proceedings of the Society for Experimental Biology and Medicine,* 92(2), 285–289.

35 de la Fuente Revenga, M., Shin, J. M., Vohra, H. Z., Hideshima, K. S., Schneck, M., Poklis, J. L., & González-Maeso, J. (2019). Fully automated head-twitch detection system for the study of 5-HT_{2A} receptor pharmacology *in vivo*. *Scientific Reports, 9*(1), 14247. https://doi.org/10.1038/s41598-019-49913-4

36 Petit-Demouliere, B., Chenu, F., & Bourin, M. (2005). Forced swimming test in mice: A review of antidepressant activity. *Psychopharmacology, 177*(3), 245–255. https://doi.org/10.1007/s00213-004-2048-7

37 PowerfulJRE. (2019, November 15). *Joe Rogan Experience #1385 – Paul Stamets* [Video]. YouTube. https://www.youtube.com/watch?v=xJ6Ym719urg

38 Beck, S. A., Barlow, C., Engel, L., & Barratt, M. J. (2025). 'Wood-lover paralysis': Describing a toxidrome with symptoms of weakness caused by some lignicolous 'wood-loving' Psilocybe mushrooms. *Toxicon, 264,* 108450. https://doi.org/10.1016/j.toxicon.2025.108450

39 Jamieson (2025). *Finding into death without inquest,* p. 12.

3 Microdosing

1 Leary, Timothy (1990). *Flashbacks: A personal and cultural history of an era.* Putnam Books, p. 253.

2 International Center for Ethnobotanical Education, Research, and Service. (2019, September 20). *San Pedro: Basic info.* https://www.iceers.org/en/basic-info/san-pedro-basic-info; Labate, B. C. (2011). Consumption of ayahuasca by children and pregnant women: Medical controversies and religious perspectives. *Journal of Psychoactive Drugs, 43*(1), 27–35. https://doi.org/10.1080/02791072.2011.566498

3 Fadiman, J. (2011). *The psychedelic explorer's guide: Safe, therapeutic, and sacred journeys*. Park Street Press.

4 Leonard, A. (2015, November 20). How LSD microdosing became the hot new business trip. *Rolling Stone*. https://www.rollingstone.com/culture/culture-news/how-lsd-microdosing-became-the-hot-new-business-trip-64961/; Glatter, R. (2015, November 27). LSD microdosing: The new job enhancer in Silicon Valley and beyond? *Forbes*. https://www.forbes.com/sites/robertglatter/2015/11/27/lsd-microdosing-the-new-job-enhancer-in-silicon-valley-and-beyond/; Solon, O. (2016, August 24). Under pressure, Silicon Valley workers turn to LSD microdosing. *Wired*. https://www.wired.com/story/lsd-microdosing-drugs-silicon-valley/

5 Solon (2016). Under pressure.

6 Polito, V, & Stevenson, R. J. (2019). A systematic study of microdosing psychedelics. *PLoS ONE, 14*(2), e0211023. https://doi.org/10.1371/journal.pone.0211023

7 Szigeti, B., Kartner, L., Blemings, A., Rosas, F., Feilding, A., Nutt, D. J., Carhart-Harris, R. L., & Erritzoe, D. (2021). Self-blinding citizen science to explore psychedelic microdosing. *eLife, 10*, e62878. https://doi.org/10.7554/eLife.62878

8 Meshkat, S., Al-Shamali, H., Perivolaris, A., Tullu, T., Zeifman, R. J., Zhang, Y., Burback, L., Winkler, O., Greenshaw, A., Husain, M. I., C Reichelt, A., Vermetten, E., Jha, M. K., Jetly, R., Loebenberg, R., & Bhat, V. (2025). Pharmacokinetics of psilocybin: A systematic review. *Pharmaceutics, 17*(4), 411. https://doi.org/10.3390/pharmaceutics17040411

9 Rutherford, B. R., Wager, T. D., & Roose, S. P. (2010). Expectancy and the treatment of depression: A review of experimental methodology and effects on patient outcome. *Current Psychiatry Reviews, 6*(1), 1–10. https://doi.org/10.2174/157340010790596571

10 Noorani, T. (2020, July 20). The Pollan Effect: Psychedelic research between world and word. *Fieldsights*. https://www.culanth.org/fieldsights/the-pollan-effect-psychedelic-research-between-world-and-word

11 Haridy, R. (2021, June 13). The problem at the heart of modern psychedelic clinical research. *New Atlas*. https://newatlas.com/science/placebo-problem-blinding-modern-psychedelic-science/

12 Olson, J. A., Suissa-Rocheleau, L., Lifshitz, M., Raz, A., & Veissière, S. P. L. (2020). Tripping on nothing: Placebo psychedelics and contextual factors. *Psychopharmacology, 237*(5), 1371–1382. https://doi.org/10.1007/s00213-020-05464-5

13 Aday, J. S., Simonsson, O., Schindler, E. A. D., & D'Souza, D. C. (2025). Addressing blinding in classic psychedelic studies with innovative active placebos. *International Journal of Neuropsychopharmacology, 28*(4), pyaf023. https://doi.org/10.1093/ijnp/pyaf023

14 Microdosing Institute. (2024, December 26). *Microdosing protocols.* https://microdosinginstitute.com/how-to/microdosing-protocols/

15 Hutten, N. R. P. W., Mason, N. L., Dolder, P. C., & Kuypers, K. P. C. (2019). Motives and side-effects of microdosing with psychedelics among users. *International Journal of Neuropsychopharmacology, 22*(7), 426–434. https://doi.org/10.1093/ijnp/pyz029

16 Carhart-Harris, R., Giribaldi, B., Watts, R., Baker-Jones, M., Murphy-Beiner, A., Murphy, R., Martell, J., Blemings, A., Erritzoe, D., & Nutt, D. J. (2021). Trial of psilocybin versus escitalopram for depression. *New England Journal of Medicine, 384*(15), 1402–1411. https://doi.org/10.1056/nejmoa2032994

17 Carhart-Harris, R. [@RCarhartHarris]. (2021, April 8). *Each day until publication at 5pm ET on 14th april, I'll give some brief about the paper …* [Thumbnail with link attached] [Post]. X. https://x.com/RCarhartHarris/status/1380049694953512960

18 Haridy, R. (2021, April 14). First head-to-head trial pits psychedelic therapy against antidepressant. *New Atlas.* https://newatlas.com/science/psychdelic-psilocybin-trial-antidepressant-comparison-study/

19 Williams, J. B., Kobak, K. A., Bech, P., Engelhardt, N., Evans, K., Lipsitz, J., Olin, J., Pearson, J., & Kalali, A. (2008). The GRID-HAMD: Standardization of the Hamilton Depression Rating Scale. *International Clinical Psychopharmacology, 23*(3), 120–129. https://doi.org/10.1097/YIC.0b013e3282f948f5

20 Daldegan-Bueno, D., Donegan, C. J., Sumner, R., Forsyth, A., Evans, W., Alshakhouri, M., Reynolds, L., Ponton, R., Smith, T., Roop, P., Hoeh, N., Allen, N., Sundram, F., Menkes, D., & Muthukumaraswamy, S. (2026). LSD microdosing in major depressive disorder: Results from an open-label trial. *Neuropharmacology, 283*, 110762. https://doi.org/10.1016/j.neuropharm.2025.110762

21 Hanka, J. (2025, November 16). *I'm still in disbelief! After so many years of clinical trials and hope for this treatment for depression …* [Thumbnail with link attached] [Post]. LinkedIn. https://www.linkedin.com/posts/justinhanka_microdosing-in-depression-trial-initial-results-ugcPost-7395932765466103808-gen0/

4 DMT

1 Much of the ayahuasca story recounted here comes from a wonderful source on the Kahpi website (https://www.kahpi.net). The site has pulled together a mass of academic and field studies on ayahuasca to create what I suggest is the most comprehensive resource on the subject: Kahpi. (2020). *1648-1768 – The first written reports of ayahuasca made by Jesuit missionaries.* Ayahuasca Timeline. https://ayahuasca-timeline.kahpi.net/ayahuasca-first-reports-jesuit-missionaries/

2 Gallimore, A. R. (2025, July 16). *Nature's strangest psychedelic is everywhere: The ever-surprising history of DMT.* Literary Hub. https://lithub.com/natures-strangest-psychedelic-is-everywhere-the-ever-

surprising-history-of-dmt/; Sheldrake, M. (2020). The 'enigma' of Richard Schultes, Amazonian hallucinogenic plants, and the limits of ethnobotany. *Social Studies of Science, 50*(3), 345–376. https://doi.org/10.1177/0306312720920362

3 Miles, B. (2015). *William S. Burroughs: A life.* Weidenfeld & Nicolson.

4 Burroughs, W. S., & Ginsberg, A. (2012). *The Yage letters.* Penguin. (Original work published 1963). Appendix 4. Without being too reductive, we can consider yagé another name for ayahuasca. The two names generally refer to similar concoctions, but yagé is used by communities indigenous to areas in Colombia, and ayahuasca is more commonly used around Peru and Brazil. Some people suggest there are slight procedural differences in the making of each brew, and the accompanying rituals are obviously different based on a variety of indigenous traditions.

5 Burroughs & Ginsberg (2012). *Yage letters,* introduction.

6 Lees, A. J. (2017). William Burroughs: Sailor of the soul. *Journal of Psychoactive Drugs, 49*(5), 385–392. https://doi.org/10.1080/02791072.2017.1357862

7 Lees (2017). *William Burroughs.*

8 Nardou, R., Sawyer, E., Song, Y. J., Wilkinson, M., Padovan-Hernandez, Y., de Deus, J. L., Wright, N., Lama, C., Faltin, S., Goff, L. A., Stein-O'Brien, G. L., & Dölen, G. (2023). Psychedelics reopen the social reward learning critical period. *Nature, 618*(7966), 790–798. https://www.nature.com/articles/s41586-023-06204-3

9 Bonomo, Y. A., Norman, A. F., Collins, L., Ross, M., Dwyer, J., Perkins, D., & Sarris, J. (2025). DMT and harmala alkaloids: an exploratory study of oral Acacia based formulations in healthy volunteers. *Frontiers in Psychiatry, 16,* 1545915. https://doi.org/10.3389/fpsyt.2025.1545915

10 Gallimore, A. R. (2025). *Death by astonishment: Confronting the mystery of the world's strangest drug.* St Martin's Press.

11 Timmermann, C., Zeifman, R. J., Erritzoe, D., Nutt, D. J., & Carhart-Harris, R. L. (2024). Effects of DMT on mental health outcomes in healthy volunteers. *Scientific Reports, 14*(1), 3097. https://doi.org/10.1038/s41598-024-53363-y

12 Strassman, R. (2001). *DMT: The spirit molecule: A doctor's revolutionary research into the biology of near-death and mystical experiences.* Park Street Press, p. 187.

13 Strassman (2001). *DMT,* p. 183.

14 Strassman (2001). *DMT,* p. 183.

15 Evans, J. (2023, September 8). Encounters with negative entities. *Ecstatic Integration.* https://www.ecstaticintegration.org/p/encounters-with-negative-entities

16 Davis, A. K., Clifton, J. M., Weaver, E. G., Hurwitz, E. S., Johnson, M. W., & Griffiths, R. R. (2020). Survey of entity encounter experiences occasioned by inhaled N,N-dimethyltryptamine: Phenomenology, interpretation, and enduring effects. *Journal of Psychopharmacology, 34*(9), 1008–1020. https://doi.org/10.1177/0269881120916143

17 Bouso, J. C., Andión, Ó., Sarris, J. J., Scheidegger, M., Tófoli, L. F., Opaleye, E. S., Schubert, V., & Perkins, D. (2022). Adverse effects of ayahuasca: Results from the Global Ayahuasca Survey. *PLOS Global Public Health, 2*(11), e0000438. https://doi.org/10.1371/journal.pgph.0000438

18 Holmstedt, B. (1965). Tryptamine derivatives in Epená, an intoxicating snuff used by some South American Indian tribes. *Archives internationales de pharmacodynamie et de therapie, 156*(2), 285–305.

19 Erspamer, V., Vitali, T., Roseghini, M., & Cei, J. M. (1967). 5-Methoxy- and 5-Hydroxyindoles in the skin of *Bufo alvarius*. *Biochemical Pharmacology, 16*(7), 1149–1164. https://doi.org/10.1016/0006-2952(67)90147-5

20 Delgrasso, A. (2024). Defining 5-MeO-DMT in historical and cultural contexts. *World Futures, 80*(2), 174–197. https://doi.org/10.1080/02604027.2024.2330255; Pollan, M. (2018). *How to change your mind: What the new science of psychedelics teaches us about consciousness, dying, addiction, depression, and transcendence*. Penguin, p. 274.

21 Lii, T. R., Smith, A. E., Flohr, J. R., Okada, R. L., Nyongesa, C. A., Cianfichi, L. J., Hack, L. M., Schatzberg, A. F., & Heifets, B. D. (2023). Randomized trial of ketamine masked by surgical anesthesia in patients with depression. *Nature Mental Health, 1*(11), 876–886. https://doi.org/10.1038/s44220-023-00140-x

22 Azmitia, E. C. (2010). Evolution of serotonin: Sunlight to suicide. In Müller, C. P., & Jacobs, B. L. (Eds.), *Handbook of Behavioral Neuroscience* (pp. 3–22). Elsevier. https://doi.org/10.1016/s1569–7339(10)70069–2

23 Jain, M. K., Gumpper, R. H., Slocum, S. T., Schmitz, G. P., Madsen, J. S., Tummino, T. A., Suomivuori, C. M., Huang, X. P., Shub, L., DiBerto, J. F., Kim, K., DeLeon, C., Krumm, B. E., Fay, J. F., Keiser, M., Hauser, A. S., Dror, R. O., Shoichet, B., Gloriam, D. E., … Roth, B. L. (2025). The polypharmacology of psychedelics reveals multiple targets for potential therapeutics. *Neuron, 113*(19), 3129–3142.e9. https://doi.org/10.1016/j.neuron.2025.06.012

24 Duman, R. S., Aghajanian, G. K., Sanacora, G., & Krystal, J. H. (2016). Synaptic plasticity and depression: New insights from stress and rapid-acting antidepressants. *Nature Medicine, 22*(3), 238–249. https://doi.org/10.1038/nm.4050

25 Li, N., Lee, B., Liu, R. J., Banasr, M., Dwyer, J. M., Iwata, M., Li, X. Y., Aghajanian, G., & Duman, R. S. (2010). mTOR-dependent synapse formation underlies the rapid antidepressant effects of NMDA antagonists. *Science, 329*(5994), 959–964. https://doi.org/10.1126/science.1190287

26 Olson, D. E. (2018). Psychoplastogens: A promising class of plasticity-promoting neurotherapeutics. *Journal of Experimental Neuroscience, 12*, 1179069518800508. https://doi.org/10.1177/1179069518800508

27 Shao, L. X., Liao, C., Gregg, I., Davoudian, P. A., Savalia, N. K., Delagarza, K., & Kwan, A. C. (2021). Psilocybin induces rapid and

persistent growth of dendritic spines in frontal cortex *in vivo*. *Neuron, 109*(16), 2535–2544.e4. https://doi.org/10.1016/j.neuron.2021.06.008; Jefferson, S. J., Gregg, I., Dibbs, M., Liao, C., Wu, H., Davoudian, P. A., Woodburn, S. C., Wehrle, P. H., Sprouse, J. S., Sherwood, A. M., Kaye, A. P., Pittenger, C., & Kwan, A. C. (2023). 5-MeO-DMT modifies innate behaviors and promotes structural neural plasticity in mice. *Neuropsychopharmacology, 48*(9), 1257–1266. https://doi.org/10.1038/s41386-023-01572-w

28 Wolff, M., Gukasyan, N., Roseman, L., & Liknaitzky, P. (2025). Reframing psychedelic regulation: Tools, not treatments. *Drug Science, Policy and Law, 11*. https://doi.org/10.1177/20503245251348272

5 MDMA

1 Switzerland has a limited-access model for psychedelic medicine. It has been running for nearly a decade and involves authorised medical practitioners using LSD, psilocybin and MDMA in clinical contexts. This model differs from the Australian model insofar as it requires each patient to get individual approval from a public health agency before treatment. In contrast, once authorised, an Australian psychiatrist can prescribe the medicines as frequently as they see fit without any specific oversight.

2 Baker, J. (2024, February 7). An Australian doctor has just made global history. This is what happened. *Sydney Morning Herald*. https://www.smh.com.au/national/an-australian-doctor-has-just-made-global-history-this-is-what-happened-20240206-p5f2v0.html

3 Schweickle, M., & Cassidy, T. (2024). Six month follow up of one of the first patients to complete MDMA-assisted therapy for PTSD outside of clinical trials in Australia: Implications for translating clinical research to clinical practice. *International Journal of Psychology, 9*(6), 28–38. https://doi.org/10.47604/ijp.3113

4 Therapeutic Goods Administration. (2023, February 3). *Notice of final decision to amend (or not amend) the current Poisons Standard – June 2022 ACMS #38 – Psilocybine and MDMA*. https://www.tga.gov.au/resources/publication/scheduling-decisions-final/notice-final-decision-amend-or-not-amend-current-poisons-standard-june-2022-acms-38-psilocybine-and-mdma

5 Haridy, R. (2023). Australia to prescribe MDMA and psilocybin for PTSD and depression in world first. *Nature, 619*, 227–228. https://doi: https://doi.org/10.1038/d41586-023-02093-8

6 Therapeutic Goods Administration. (2026). *FOI 26–2560* [FOI request/report]. https://www.tga.gov.au/sites/default/files/2026-02/FOI%2026-2560.PDF

7 Passie, T.(2023). *The history of MDMA*. Oxford University Press.

8 van der Kolk, B. (2014). *The body keeps the score: Brain, mind, and body in the healing of trauma*. Penguin.

9 The supposition that 'everything is trauma' has been countered by an idea known as 'concept creep', coined by University of Melbourne psychology

professor Nick Haslam. The suggestion is that we have stretched the boundary of clinical pathologies such as abuse and trauma so far that all meaning of the terms has been diluted. According to Haslam, everyday scenarios are now being framed as PTSD-like traumas, subsequently pathologising every form as adversity in life, from romantic break-ups to minor illness. Some research suggests framing moderate adversity as trauma can weaken our capacity to cope and undermine general psychological resilience. See Haslam, N. (2016). Concept creep: Psychology's expanding concepts of harm and pathology. *Psychological Inquiry, 27*(1), 1–17. https://doi.org/10.1080/1047840X.2016.1082418; Jones, P. J., & McNally, R. J. (2022). Does broadening one's concept of trauma undermine resilience? *Psychological Trauma: Theory, Research, Practice, and Policy, 14*(S1), S131–S139. https://doi.org/10.1037/tra0001063

10 Cohen, S. (1964). *The beyond within: The LSD story.* Atheneum, pp. 182–183.

11 Langlitz, N., & Gearin, A. K. (2024). Psychedelic therapy as form of life. *Neuroethics, 17*(1), Article 14. https://doi.org/10.1007/s12152-024-09550-9

12 Cuijpers, P. (2017). Four decades of outcome research on psychotherapies for adult depression: An overview of a series of meta-analyses. *Canadian Psychology/Psychologie Canadienne, 58*(1), 7–19. https://doi.org/10.1037/cap0000096

13 Mithoefer, M. C. (2017). *A manual for MDMA-assisted psychotherapy in the treatment of posttraumatic stress disorder.* Version 8.1. Multidisciplinary Association for Psychedelic Studies. https://maps.org/wp-content/uploads/2022/05/MDMA-Assisted-Psychotherapy-Treatment-Manual-V8.1-22AUG2017.pdf

14 Griffin, A. (2025). *The tell: A memoir.* Random House, p. 75.

15 Rosman, K., & Egan, E. (2025, September 24). The billionaire, the psychedelics and the best-selling memoir. *New York Times.* https://www.nytimes.com/2025/09/24/nyregion/amy-griffin-memoir-psychedelic-drugs.html

16 Rosman & Egan. (2025). *The billionaire, the psychedelics.*

17 Busch, A. K., & Johnson, W. C. (1950). L.S.D. 25 as an aid in psychotherapy; preliminary report of a new drug. *Diseases of the Nervous System, 11*(8), 241–243.

18 Sandison, R. A., Spencer, A. M., & Whitelaw, J. D. A. (1954). The therapeutic value of lysergic acid diethylamide in mental illness. *Journal of Mental Science, 100*(419), 491–507. https://doi.org/10.1192/bjp.100.419.491

19 Smith, M., & Pazdar, L. (1980) *Michelle remembers.* St Martin's Press, p. 13.

20 Goleman, D. (1994, October 31). Proof lacking for ritual abuse by satanists. *New York Times.* https://www.nytimes.com/1994/10/31/us/proof-lacking-for-ritual-abuse-by-satanists.html

21 Crews, F. (1995). *The memory wars: Freud's legacy in dispute.* New York Review of Books.

22 Loftus, E. F., & Ketcham, K. (1994). *The myth of repressed memory: False memories and allegations of sexual abuse.* St Martin's Press.

23 Kezelman, C. (2010). *Innocence revisited: A tale in parts.* JoJo Publishing.

24 Guilliatt, R. (2017, September 30). Through the past, darkly. *Weekend Australian Magazine,* p. 14. https://www.theaustralian.com.au

25 Stavropoulos, P. A., & Kezelman, C. A. (2018). *The truth of memory and the memory of truth: Different types of memory and the significance of trauma.* Blue Knot Foundation.

26 Over recent years there has been a relatively widespread acceptance of the practice of EMDR among clinical psychologists despite some vocal critics claiming it to be a pseudoscience. Arguments against EMDR suggest the practice is no different to exposure-based cognitive behavioural therapy and the distinctive features such as eye movements are irrelevant to the results. The most recent systematic review on EMDR, published in 2024, backed this criticism up, finding it to be no more effective than other successful PTSD treatments including relaxation therapy, emotional freedom technique, and trauma-focused cognitive behavioural psychotherapies: Wright, S. L., Karyotaki, E., Cuijpers, P., Bisson, J., Papola, D., Witteveen, A., Suliman, S., Spies, G., Ahmadi, K., Capezzani, L., Carletto, S., Karatzias, T., Kullack, C., Laugharne, J., Lee, C. W., Nijdam, M. J., Olff, M., Ostacoli, L., Seedat, S., & Sijbrandij, M. (2024). EMDR *v.* other psychological therapies for PTSD: A systematic review and individual participant data meta-analysis. *Psychological Medicine,* 54(8), 1580–1588. https://doi.org/10.1017/S0033291723003446

27 Hall, W. (2021, September 25). Ending the silence around psychedelic therapy abuse. *Mad in America.* https://www.madinamerica.com/2021/09/ending-silence-psychedelic-therapy-abuse/

28 MacBride, K. (2021, November 17). 'Aharon said it was healing'. *Inverse.* https://www.inverse.com/mind-body/grossbard-bourzat-psychedelic-assisted-therapy-abuse

29 Holotropic breathwork is another controversial therapeutic technique often used in modern psychedelic medicine and labelled by some as pseudoscience. It was developed by psychiatrist Stan Grof, and he describes the technique this way: 'What happens in this process is that faster breathing, extended for a long period of time, changes the person's chemistry so that blocked physical and emotional energies, which are associated with various traumatic memories, are released and become available for peripheral discharge and processing. This makes it possible for the previously repressed content of these memories to emerge into consciousness and be integrated.' Grof, S. (2019). *The way of the psychonaut: Encyclopedia for inner journeys* (Vol. 1). Multidisciplinary Association for Psychedelic Studies, p. 389.

30 Mithoefer (2017), *Manual for MDMA-assisted psychotherapy.*

31 Mithoefer (2017), *Manual for MDMA-assisted psychotherapy*, p. 34.
32 Mithoefer (2017), *Manual for MDMA-assisted psychotherapy*, p. 26.
33 Mithoefer (2017), *Manual for MDMA-assisted psychotherapy*, p. 31.
34 Mithoefer (2017), *Manual for MDMA-assisted psychotherapy*, p. 11.
35 Grof, S. (1976). *Realms of the human unconscious: Observations from LSD research*. Dutton, p. 216
36 Greer, E. (1985). Using MDMA in psychotherapy. *Advances*, 2(2), 57–59.
37 Grof (2019). *The way of the psychonaut* (Vol. 1), p. 20.
38 Mithoefer, *Manual for MDMA-assisted psychotherapy*, pp. 16–17.
39 Grof, S. (2019). *The way of the psychonaut: Encyclopedia for inner journeys* (Vol. 2). Multidisciplinary Association for Psychedelic Studies, p. 333.
40 Grof (2019). *The way of the psychonaut* (Vol. 1), p. 328.
41 Doblin, R. (2014). Stanislav Grof's contributions to FDA drug development research with psychedelics. In *Expanding and reenchanting the psyche: The pioneering thought of Stanislav Grof*. California Institute of Integral Studies. https://digitalcommons.ciis.edu/stanislavgrof2014/12
42 Royal Australian and New Zealand College of Psychiatrists. (2025, June). *Psychedelic training framework for psychiatrists*. https://www.ranzcp.org/getmedia/b76842a8–487f-49f5-aa1f-000f8cba550f/Psychedelics-Training-Framework-June-2025.pdf
43 Interlandi, J. (2014, May 22). A revolutionary approach to treating PTSD. *New York Times*. https://www.nytimes.com/2014/05/25/magazine/a-revolutionary-approach-to-treating-ptsd.html
44 van der Kolk (2014). *Body keeps the score*, pp. 223–224.
45 BioMedical Institute of Yoga and Meditation. (2023). *200PAP Graduate Certificate in Psychedelic-Assisted PsychoSomatic Therapy*. https://biyome.com.au/course-pages/200pap/
46 Curtis, A. (Producer & Writer). (2002). There is a policeman inside all our heads: He must be destroyed (Episode 3) [TV series episode]. *The century of the self*. BBC; RDF Media.
47 Curtis (2002). There is a policeman inside all our heads.
48 Passie (2023). *History of MDMA*.
49 Marin, P. (1975, October). The new narcissism. *Harper's Magazine*, pp. 45–56.

6 Futures

1 Noorani, T. (2020). Making psychedelics into medicines: The politics and paradoxes of medicalization. *Journal of Psychedelic Studies*, 4(1), 34–39. https://doi.org/10.1556/2054.2019.018
2 For example: Cox, D. (2024, September 11). *What Western medicine can learn from the ancient history of psychedelics*. BBC, https://www.bbc.com/future/article/20240910-the-ancient-history-behind-healing-trauma-with-psychedelics; Carhart-Harris, R. L., & Goodwin, G. M. (2017). The therapeutic potential of psychedelic drugs: Past, present, and future. *Neuropsychopharmacology*, 42(11), 2105–2113. https://doi.org/10.1038/npp.2017.84

3 Singh, M. (2025). *Shamanism: The timeless religion*. Knopf.

4 An example of this common characterisation appears a 2019 Q&A with Charles Grob, one of the leading figures in modern psychedelic research, who says: 'In shamanism, psychedelics are taken only in ceremony under the guidance and supervision of the shaman, or the spiritual leader of the community. The shaman would administer these compounds only for very clear circumscribed reasons, such as an initiation rite or a healing ceremony to address individuals with severe medical or psychological problems. In the shamanic world, these compounds are never taken for frivolous reasons. That would be absolutely taboo.' In Goop, *Shamanism and psychedelics – The science behind it*. (2019, January 10). https://goop.com/wellness/health/the-science-and-shamanism-of-psychedelics/

5 Singh (2025). *Shamanism*, ch. 11.

6 Australia New Zealand Clinical Trials Registry. (2025, July 28). *Efficacy and safety of fly-in-fly-out (FIFO) model of psilocybin-assisted therapy (PAT) for major depressive disorder (MDD)*. Registration no. ACTRN12625000799459. https://anzctr.org.au/Trial/Registration/TrialReview.aspx?id=389703

7 Haridy, R. (2022, July 26). Meet two researchers bringing VR to psychedelic therapy. *New Atlas*. https://newatlas.com/science/vr-psychedelic-therapy-virtual-reality-enosis/

8 Tramacchi, D. (2004). Entheogenic dance ecstasis: Cross-cultural contexts. In St John, G. (Ed.), *Rave culture and religion* (pp. 165–182). Routledge.

9 Biwer, M. E., Álvarez, W. Y., Bautista, S. L., & Jennings, J. (2022). Hallucinogens, alcohol and shifting leadership strategies in the ancient Peruvian Andes. *Antiquity*, 96(385), 142–158. https://doi.org/10.15184/aqy.2021.177

10 de Borhegyi, C., & de Borhegyi-Forrest, S. (2015). Mushroom intoxication in Mesoamerica. In Wexler, P. (Ed.), *History of toxicology and environmental health: Toxicology in antiquity, volume II* (pp. 104–115). Academic Press, p. 109.

11 Pazzanese, C. (2024, November 1). 'I wanted to make a difference in America.' *Harvard Gazette*. https://news.harvard.edu/gazette/story/2024/11/robert-putnam-wants-us-to-stop-bowling-alone/

12 Putnam, R. D. (1995). Bowling alone: America's declining social capital. *Journal of Democracy*, 6(1), 65–78, https://doi.org/10.1353/jod.1995.0002; Putnam, R. D. (2000). *Bowling alone: The collapse and revival of American community*. Simon & Schuster.

13 Putnam, R. D., Leonardi, R., & Nanetti, R. (1993). *Making democracy work: Civic traditions in modern Italy*. Princeton University Press, p. 115.

14 Leigh, A. (2011). *Disconnected*. NewSouth Publishing, p. 129.

15 Thompson, D. (2025, February). The anti-social century. *The Atlantic*. https://www.theatlantic.com/magazine/archive/2025/02/american-loneliness-personality-politics/681091/

16 WHO Commission on Social Connection. (2025). *From loneliness to social connection – charting a path to healthier societies: Report of the WHO Commission on Social Connection*. World Health Organization. https://www.who.int/groups/commission-on-social-connection/report

17 Swann, W. B., Jetten, J., Gómez, A., Whitehouse, H., & Bastian, B. (2012). When group membership gets personal: A theory of identity fusion. *Psychological Review, 119*(3), 441–456. https://doi.org/10.1037/a0028589

18 Shapiro, N., & Kirksey, E. (2017). Chemo-ethnography: An introduction. *Cultural Anthropology, 32*(4), 481–493. https://doi.org/10.14506/ca32.4.01

19 Anderson, B. T., Danforth, A., Daroff, P. R., Stauffer, C., Ekman, E., Agin-Liebes, G., Trope, A., Boden, M. T., Dilley, P. J., Mitchell, J., & Woolley, J. (2020). Psilocybin-assisted group therapy for demoralized older long-term AIDS survivor men: An open-label safety and feasibility pilot study. *EClinicalMedicine, 27*, 100538.

20 Brown, M. (2018, March). Compassionate community project. *Resurgence & Ecologist*. https://www.resurgence.org/magazine/article5039-compassionate-community-project.html

21 Beyond Tomorrow Clips. (2025, November 27). *My first mushroom trip was the most important moment of my life – Christian Angermayer* [Video]. YouTube. https://www.youtube.com/watch?v=JLZPte5U_Yk. Angermayer often makes clear, as if it makes some kind of difference, that this experience was entirely 'legal', as some islands in the Caribbean have legalised private uses of psilocybin-containing mushrooms.

PSYCHEDELIC BOOK CLUB

If you have read this far and feel like your psychedelic curiosity needs a little more tickling, here is a further reading list. This is a list of books that are (mostly) off the beaten path in terms of the standard psychedelic reader. I can wholeheartedly recommend each and every one of these. And if you read them all back to back, I am pretty sure the machine elves will come to you without the need of DMT.

Andy Roberts, *Albion Dreaming: A Popular History of LSD in London,* Psychedelic Press, 2025
I'm always a fan of alternative history books. There have been dozens of books telling the story of LSD in North America but there is only one telling the tale of how it swept the United Kingdom. Well researched, and updated in 2025.

Mike Jay, *Psychonauts: Drugs and the Making of the Modern Mind,* Yale University Press, 2023
One of those books that can single-handedly change your perception of history. Jay traces a history of drug experimentation by artists and writers, from nitrous oxide huffing in the early 19th century to Freud and his cocaine habit. This is the first psychedelic history book I recommend to anyone and everyone who will listen.

Aldous Huxley, *The Doors of Perception,* Chatto & Windus, 1954
A classic, but it's here for a reason. I studiously avoided filling this book up with me trying to use all my fancy words describing what a psychedelic experience feels like. I've read thousands of trip reports and they are almost always boring. This book, however, is probably the best, most lucid writing describing the experience of tripping I have ever encountered. Huxley nailed it 70 years ago. No one else needs to try to do it anymore.

Erika Dyck et al. (Eds), *Women and Psychedelics: Uncovering Invisible Voices,* Synergetic Press, 2024
You may have noticed how male-centred the modern story of psychedelics is. It's a powerfully patriarchal narrative and this book is a crucial corrective centring numerous female voices in often familiar stories. A wildly important book that tells a number of untold stories.

Terence McKenna and Dennis McKenna, *The Invisible Landscape: Mind, Hallucinogens, and the I Ching,* The Seabury Press, 1975
If you wanna go direct to the source, track down the first McKenna book. Years before he went stoned ape with the well-known *Food of the Gods,* this was the book that chronicled the real weird psychedelic stuff that went down in the Amazon when these two brothers went deep into the heart of darkness to find a truth. This is the real stuff.

Andrew R Gallimore, *Death by Astonishment: Confronting the Mystery of the World's Strangest Drug,* St Martin's Press, 2025
This certainly isn't DMT expert Andrew Gallimore's most out-there book (that award goes to *Reality Switch Technologies*) but it is the most comprehensive story of DMT you will find. Covers all the bases from history to hard science, and also crosses over into weirdness with some of Gallimore's ideas about how this drug may actually be sending people into other dimensions.

Alex Gearin, *Global Ayahuasca: Wondrous Visions and Modern Worlds,* Stanford University Press, 2024
Australian anthropologist Alex Gearin presents an incredibly provocative portrait of ayahuasca use around the world. The chunk of this book that delves into the way ayahuasca is used in middle-class urban China is absolutely incredible. A head-spinning insight into the ways this traditional psychedelic brew has been incorporated into 21st-century cultures around the world.

Alexander Shulgin and Ann Shulgin, *PiHKAL: A Chemical Love Story,* Transform Press, 1991, and *TiHKAL: The Continuation,* Transform Press, 1997
Over the course of the 1960s, '70s and '80s, Alexander Shulgin created scores of new psychedelic molecules. And he studiously tested them

all on himself. These two books are the result of a lifetime of chemical experimentation. Each combines fictionalised autobiography with dozens of chemical recipes for new drugs. Some of these drugs are just now being explored as medicines in the modern psychedelic renaissance. These two books are like bibles for hard-head psychonauts.

Douglas Rushkoff, *Survival of the Richest*, Scribe, 2023
In the early 1990s, Rushkoff was hanging out with Tim Leary and writing about the techno-rave scene in Los Angeles. Now he has seen drugs and technology come full circle. This book is a prescient take on why things are how they are now. The internet is like acid, Rushkoff says, and we're in the middle of a bad trip.

Carl Hart, *Drug Use For Grown-ups: Chasing Liberty in the Land of Fear*, Penguin, 2021
A provocative book arguing for total personal liberty when it comes to drug use. Hart's book is not perfect (he occasionally twists evidence to fit his arguments) but it's a powerful thought experiment that takes all drug use and asks whether the way we are doing things is the best way.

ACKNOWLEDGEMENTS

At the point I was finishing writing this book, I read a wonderful article by Tabitha Carvan titled 'The Unexpected Poetry of PhD Acknowledgements'. Carvan waded through hundreds and hundreds of acknowledgement pages in science theses, highlighting how this often overlooked part of a thesis can contain the most meaningful and important writing by the author. Carvan also discussed how all acknowledgements seem formulaic, but despite the formula there were powerful stories behind every comment.

This rang profoundly true to me as I sat down to think about how to thank all those who helped bring this book to life. The words I put down here feel generic and insufficient but there is no other way to say something so simple and straightforward. These are the people who made this book happen.

At this top I must recognise all the work done for decades by those in the psychedelic underground. The phrase 'standing on the shoulders of giants' may be overused but it's apt in this context. Saying Australia's psychedelic renaissance kicked off in 2010 is of course a totally arbitrary pin on a calendar. There are tales of incredible people doing incredible things here in Australia with psychedelics for decades preceding that point.

Most of those who persevered in the shadows cannot tell their stories due to lingering punitive drug laws, but they must be recognised and celebrated. You know who you are. Thanks for talking to me, trusting me and sharing information. This includes all the WTF crew, plus special mention to DL, RS, LV, TW and Myz Guidance.

This is also the spot where I'll shout out all the humans who are still reading, writing and thinking. Absolutely no AI was used in the creation of this book. No journals summarised, no text 'punched up'. Everything you have read was thought by me and written word for word by me. So everything that annoyed you is 100 per cent my fault.

At the very beginning of this whole thing I called two people to ask their thoughts on the project: Jonathan Carmichael and Martin Williams, both key figures in Entheogenesis Australis. To pull off an investigation into such an insular community I'd need to know if people were going to talk to me. Connection with contacts and backing from both Jonathan and Martin were crucial and I can confidently say this book wouldn't exist without their enthusiastic support. In general, the entire EGA community has been an incredible resource. My eternal gratitude to the hundreds of people who keep that volunteer organisation alive.

I'm in debt to Megan Lomax-Whitaker for her generous time talking to me and sharing her research on psychedelic history in Australia. Her work delving into the Victorian Department of Health archives has pieced together the only robust account of psychedelic medicine in Australia we have. Across several conversations we both were struck with the many parallels between the current world of emerging psychedelic medicine and the story of the same in the 1960s.

Of course eternal gratitude to Evelyn and Vivien for sharing their historic psychedelic stories. And on the modern history tip, I'm grateful to Marg Ross for always being so open to many chats. Also so important to this final product were all the conversations with Nigel Strauss, Monica Schweickle, Ariana Elias, Steve Bright, Paul Liknaitzky, Gill Bedi, Daniel Perkins, Sam Douglas, Tehseen Noorani and every other clinician or researcher who chatted with me off the record.

All the mushroom people require particular acknowledgement. Caine Barlow, Simon Beck, Alistair McTaggart and others patiently explained complicated things to me, often many times over. And I must mention 'Kay' – thank you for sharing a story that was hard to tell. I hope we have got the message of wood-lover paralysis right.

The entire microdosing chapter is thanks to Vince Polito for trusting and allowing me into his clinical trial space. Sam Banister helped me understand the weird pharmacology of these drugs and showed me what a modern psychedelic lab looks like. Richard Guilliatt shared so much of his journalistic work on the history of recovered-memory science in Australia. Kayla Greenstien spent an exorbitant amount of time talking me through her experiences with psychedelic ethics.

A whole host of other people also require recognition, not because they are in the book but because they helped shape the stories, frequently listening to me rant about things. Sam-I-Am: thanks for reading a chapter when I had an emergency freak-out. Monica Barratt and Stu Hatton: thanks for doing the big review read and offering me some of the first encouraging words about the final product.

Emma Driver, editor extraordinaire, thanks for making all this read good and homing in on all the writerly crutches I lean on. I'm sure you'll want to cut my use of the phrase 'editor extraordinaire' but I think I get full control over this part – yeah, this should be cut, you're right. And Harriet McInerney from NewSouth Publishing, thanks most of all for poking me to write the book in the first place and encouraging me to loosen up as I wrote it. Your gentle nudging made this book so much better than it would've been without your advice.

The Science Journalists Association of Australia has been a rock of support for all my journalistic goals for several years now. Thanks Bianca Nogrady and Jackson Ryan, and also a massive chunk of travel funding came from a travel grant that I will forever be grateful for. Creative Victoria also generously supported the writing of this book with a Creative Projects Fund grant. Long may our government and institutions support book-writing and the arts.

I could almost start thanking everyone in my life as this book genuinely is the product of everything that has led me to now.

But most importantly I need to acknowledge my family for supporting me through everything. Mum, Anna and Marlow. You are the best people in the world. You made this.

Printed and bound by CPI Group (UK) Ltd, Croydon, CR0 4YY

07/10/2026

14977326-0001